KT-155-599

What's The Alternative?

Hazel Courteney

Infinity Press
P.O Box 4629,
Edgbaston,
Birmingham, B15 3TW

© 1995 Hazel Courteney

First Edition September 1995
Reprinted and revised edition November 1995
Reprinted February 1996

ISBN 0-9526122-0-8

Printed by Bath Press
Lower Bristol Road, Bath, BA2 3BL

For Stuart and Victoria.

Acknowledgements

I would like to sincerely thank all the dedicated practitioners who have given so much of their time and energy helping with my research over the past two years. Especially Dr John Stirling, Dr John Briffa, Tricia Sabine, Gareth Zeal, Rhaya Jordan, Celia Wright, Angela Dowden and Rohit Mehta.

Thanks to my wonderful doctor, Brian McGreevy for his understanding and support.

To my personal assistant Lindsey Ross-Jarrett, for her endless patience, sound advice and hard work.

Special thanks to my dear friend Kathryn Marsden, who has always been there for me.

To Norma Rhys-Davies, who knows why.

To my husband Stuart for his saintly patience and support.

Contents

Foreword

Ten years ago alternative medicine and therapies were considered by the majority to be quackery, in certain circles it is still so perceived. I find this strange when one considers that alternative treatments in the form of herbs and spices, along with therapies like acupuncture have been practised for over two thousand years.

I became involved with complementary medicine and therapies approximately nine years ago when I started to suffer from severe migraines. A friend suggested I consult Gudrun Jonsson, a Biopath, who works with dietary changes, vitamins and minerals plus homeopathy to help restore good health. She suggested various herbal remedies along with a change of diet and certain supplements. Also I was advised to drink copious amounts of hot water which contained an infusion of ginger root. Within a short period of time, I suffered fewer migraines and my weight went right down and balanced out.

There are also many qualified doctors who now use complementary medicines. Over the years Dr Mary Loveday, an allergist and clinical ecologist, has prescribed natural products along with homeopathic remedies for myself and my children, which have helped enormously with various ailments like allergies which all children suffer from time to time.

I often use the homeopathic remedy Arnica for my children when they fall or shock themselves as it calms the nervous system. I like using homeopathy for their coughs and colds, otherwise during the winter terms they would be permanently on antibiotics, which they have taken if the bug has been a severe one. I am not in any way against orthodox treatments and medicines which I know daily save thousands of lives, I simply prefer natural remedies whenever possible.

What I do notice is that when long term use of drugs has been necessary, many people suffer dreadful side effects and they are openly seeking alternative ways to become and remain healthy by alternative means.

Many in the medical profession, like Dr Loveday, are now realising that so many complementary therapies are of enormous benefit to their patients. Perhaps the time has come for more doctors and complementary practitioners to work side by side and offer integrated therapies to their patients.

In this book Hazel has given specific remedies which, while I cannot take responsibility for the results, should help an enormous number of people.

I sincerely hope that you will find all the answers you are seeking in the pages that follow. A great deal of thought and research has gone into the suggested remedies which have worked for thousands of people.

I wish you well on your journey to renewed health.

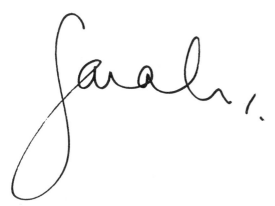

Her Royal Highness The Duchess of York

Why I wrote this book

Last year in the UK alone, 23 million prescriptions were dispensed for arthritis related diseases and 14 million for sedatives and anti depressants; not to mention the millions of over-the-counter drugs purchased daily. To what end? Often, only temporary relief from the symptoms, rarely a cure for the root of the problem. Daily, so many people suffer dreadful side effects from these drugs - skin disorders and hormone imbalance from steroids, intestinal problems and stomach ulcers from too many pain killers and allergic reactions to antibiotics; all of which have adverse effects on our natural immune systems.

When there is such an enormous amount of information available to us all about health and well-being in magazines, newspapers and on TV programmes, why do so many people continue to ignore the evidence, resulting in an ever increasing spiral of deteriorating health? I believe it's because most people are simply not open to new ideas. They are so accustomed to their parents, doctors, welfare services, hospitals and governments taking care of them and making their decisions for them that they have never given a thought to the concept of being able to help themselves. On many occasions I have interviewed people who complain about the lack of information relating to their condition that is being made available to them by their doctor. A great majority are truly shocked when I suggest that they are capable of finding alternative therapies and medicines to aid their recovery. Furthermore, I am a firm believer in the body's ability to heal itself; all it needs are the right tools for the job.

Alternatives do work for millions of people - but often doctors have little or no knowledge of alternative medicines and therapies. To be fair, many doctors are stretched to the limit, often working an exhausting schedule under tremendous pressure. Even if this were not the case, there remains the fact that in the course of five years of medical studies, they generally receive only a few hours of nutritional training. So how can we expect our family doctor to know much about vitamins, minerals, herbs, homeopathy or any other alternative treatments? They have enough trouble keeping pace with the constant flow of new products continually being sent to them by the pharmaceutical companies, who are all to eager to increase their market share in the lucrative prescription drug market.

Thankfully for all of us, the winds of change are at last beginning to blow in an alternative direction. Here and there, doctors are openly using and being trained in alternative methods of medicine. In many cases, because their own patients are demanding a change. Some people are actually asking their doctor questions about the side effects of drugs and are suggesting natural remedies which they have discovered are beneficial to their health. People everywhere are sick of being sick.

These days, in certain selective practices around the UK, you will find osteopaths, homeopaths, counsellors, nutritionists and occasionally even spiritual healers. Increasingly, more and more local health authorities are offering alternative therapies on the National Health. In fact, some doctors now openly admit that conventional medicine and alternative therapies can work in tandem for the well being of their patients, whilst many others are still afraid to speak out in favour of alternatives for fear of being labelled cranks.

Over the course of the past few years I have met, interviewed and received thousands of letters from people who have succeeded in changing their habits and discovered alternative ways of healing themselves. Some had eczema or psoriasis, others had heart disorders or arthritis; there were cases involving chronic fatigue syndrome and depression; while many more had suffered and survived through life threatening illnesses like cancer. Now, thanks entirely to sheer determination in their search for answers, most of these people are getting well. Many of them found out about alternative therapies through friends, some by investigating and inquiring about the specifics of their condition, others by having their interest awakened by an article they happened to read in a newspaper or magazine. Ultimately they were all willing to try something new, and over time they were able to wean themselves off prescription drugs, in some cases with the approval of their doctors. I believe this will be the medical science of the future - a comprehensive service to the patient in which both alternative and conventional treatments are integrated for the benefit of us all.

I am not opposed to conventional medicine, and would not advocate the abolition of prescription drugs, many of which are invaluable for savings lives. Yet so many doctors and pharmaceutical companies dismiss out of hand any and all alternative therapies. Although it is wise to view any new form of treatment with a healthy scepticism, the same goes for any treatment suggested by a doctor, who may be more inclined to prescribe drugs to deal with the symptoms than to look for the root cause of an illness.

I have been fascinated with alternative ideas for most of my life, and for the past five years I have researched alternative remedies and therapies in depth and felt a desperate need to share this knowledge with others. I started to write newspaper and magazine articles about what I had learned and they proved very popular with the readers. Since March 1994, when my weekly column first appeared in The Daily Mail, I have received many thousands of letters from readers all over the country as well as many from overseas and made a point of reading each one personally. They were answered only after careful research and consultation with doctors, nutritionists and various specialists.

No one knows all the answers, but I have been fortunate enough to discover some helpful hints that I think are worth sharing. I have taken great care to outline specific treatments for specific ailments; which supplements to take and where to buy them, in order to make the process as easy as possible. My sole purpose is to help as many people as possible to benefit from the knowledge of my experience. The path you choose to pursue is yours, I merely want to help you find your way.

You can improve the condition of your health and well-being, beginning today. If you are suffering from ill-health, you can begin to turn that around. If you are fortunate enough to enjoy good health, you can make it even better. I say this with confidence even though I don't know you. I do know that you are reading these words and as you continue to read this book you will be finding out about new treatments and medicines that you can use today and every day to improve your health and get more out of your life.

I hope you will find some useful answers in this book. I have done my best to include most of the advice and remedies which have come my way over the years and which have proved to be helpful in practice.

The inspiration for this book came from all the wonderful and thought provoking letters which have been sent to me by the readers of my column. To all of you out there who are suffering from ill health, I wish you luck on your road to recovery.

Hazel Courteney

About Vitamins and Supplements

I feel the need to explain why it is necessary to take daily vitamins in order to remain healthy on a long term basis. Your body must have vitamins and minerals in order to live, but your body cannot produce them. Therefore you must either obtain vitamins and minerals from your diet - or take supplements. But is it possible to still eat a healthy balanced diet in today's world? A century ago, there were no pesticides sprayed on our crops, nor any of the 3,500 chemical preservatives and additives found in our food today. In country areas the air was cleaner, acid rain did not pollute our crops. There are over 3,000 chemicals in the air, from the lead in car exhaust fumes, cadmium from cigarettes to mercury in pesticides. These alone cause hyperactivity, aggressive behaviour, memory loss, confusion and cancer.

With the limited exception of a few farmers who grow organic fruit and vegetables, the majority of produce we eat today has lost much of it's nutritional value. Many of us eat convenience foods as we live at such a fast pace. Most pre-packaged food loses all it's vitamin content in the packaging and reheating process - not to mention the amount of added preservatives. Even when we think we are eating a healthy balanced diet, often we are not. Vegetables and fruit are covered in pesticides. It is estimated that each and every one of us has up to a gallon of pesticides and herbicides sprayed on the fruit and vegetables we eat in a year, as well as eating 12lbs of food additives. Vegetables stored in a fridge for three days lose 50% of the vitamin content, cooking often destroys the rest.

Sulphur from acid rain destroys the mineral selenium in our soil. In Bulgaria where the soil is rich in selenium, there is a low incidence of heart disease. In Finland and Denmark it is added to the soil. In the UK, heart disease, mental problems and cancer are reaching epidemic proportions. One in three people will at some time contract cancer, one in ten will have mental health problems.

The air and food are riddled with free radicals which damage our cells causing early ageing and disease. Antioxidants are the vitamins and minerals we need to take every day of our lives to protect our health, vitamins and minerals are NOT drugs. To my mind, many diseases can be prevented by changing our diets and taking supplements. The Health Service which is on the verge of collapse could be saved. We could die of old age, but live happier, healthier, more productive lives, if we are willing to take responsibility for our health from now on. Health is wealth.

Many people argue that they do eat a balanced diet and therefore do not need vitamins. But imagine a pregnant woman who is told to eat broccoli as a source of folic acid, which helps prevent birth defects. To obtain the recommended intake she would need to eat 5lbs of broccoli daily! We all need at least 1gram of vitamin C daily - this would mean eating fifteen oranges. Is it not simpler to guarantee the correct dose by simply taking a vitamin pill?

I am well aware that vitamins should never be used as a substitute for a healthy balanced diet, but they can be of enormous benefit if used properly. Before reading the hints section, here are a few tips on how best to use your supplements for optimum benefits.

• Read instructions on labels carefully and never exceed the maximum dose.

• Many vitamins and supplements currently on the market have less than optimum quantities of beneficial ingredients. As it happens, you get much better value by purchasing the best quality vitamins and supplements because their individual content is far higher.

• Most vitamins have a good shelf life but will cease to be effective if you keep them for too long. Be aware of sell-by dates and always keep your vitamins in a cool, dry place - never expose them to direct sunlight.

• Vitamins taken regularly have a progressive affect and taken in the long term almost always produce beneficial effects. Don't expect miracles in a week. If you start a course of vitamins, minerals or any supplements give them at least three months in order to see the benefits. Any changes in your health will be very subtle.

The Codes - How to use this book

Throughout this book I have used codes to identify specific brands. If no code or other details are mentioned then the supplements should be available at any good health store.

BC Bio Care. Lakeside, 180, Lifford Lane, Kings Norton, Birmingham. B30 3NT. Tel. 0121 433 3727. Fax. 0121 433 3879.

BLK Blackmores Ltd, 37 Rothschild Road, London. W4 5HT. Tel. 0181 987 8640. Fax. 0181 987 8641.

FSC The Health and Diet Company, Europa Park, Stone Clough Road, Radclliffe, Manchester. M26 1GG. Tel. 01204 707420. Fax. 01204 792238.

HN Higher Nature Ltd, The Nutrition Centre, Burwash Common, East Sussex. TN 19 7LX. Tel. 01435 882 880. Fax. 01435 883 720.

LGF Larkhall Green Farm, 225, Putney Bridge Road, London. SW15 2PY. Tel. 0181 874 1130. Fax. 0181 871 0066.

NC The Nutri Centre, The Hale Clinic, 7, Park Crescent, London. N1N 3HE. Tel. 0171 436 5122. Fax. 0171 436 5171.

Q Quest Vitamins. 8, Venture Way, Aston Science Park, Birmingham. B74AP. Tel. 0121 359 0056. Fax. 0121 359 0313.

For all other addresses and details see the index on page 148

Author's Note

No-one is more aware than myself as to the hundreds of alternative supplements now available in the UK. In this book I have suggested several specific brands which I have used regularly for some years. If I tried to mention every brand by name, the book would not be an easy to read book of hints, but a lengthy encyclopedia. My personal preference for specific brands in no way infers that they are better or more beneficial than others on the market. If you have specific brands you know and trust, check to see if they have similar supplements to those recommended in the hints section.

Some people have reactions to certain supplements. This is usually caused by an allergy to one of the ingredients contained in the supplement, not to the nutrients themselves which we all need. Better quality brands use hypo allergenic ingredients, therefore choose high quality brands.

Vitamin supplements are intended to prevent deficiency and thereby strengthen the body. This book is not intended as a substitute for conventional medical counselling. Never stop taking prescribed medicine without first consulting your doctor. In matters that pertain to your health, always see your doctor.

ACID STOMACH (see also Indigestion and Low Stomach Acid)

During an average lifetime, 100 tons of food passes through the digestive tract and 300 litres of digestive juices are produced by the body to break it down; it's no wonder so many people end up with acid stomach, indigestion, and heartburn. Most of us eat far too many acid forming foods like bread, cakes, biscuits, sugar, meat, fish, pasta, coffee, milk and alcohol. We often eat too much food during one meal and combine foods which fight each other inside the stomach.

DIET

Eat more alkaline forming foods such as fresh fruit, vegetables and salad. Replace dairy products made from cow's milk with non-dairy soya products. Raw vegetables contain important enzymes which help digestion. If you find raw vegetables hard to digest then buy a vegetable juicer and make a daily mix of any fresh vegetables. My favourite is a blend of carrot, apple, root ginger, celery and spinach. Drink immediately to gain the full benefits of all the vitamins and live enzymes. Limit alcohol intake and stop smoking as these aggravate an acid stomach.

SUPPLEMENTS

Sea Plasma, to re-alkalise the system.
Citrase, containing calcium and magnesium, which alkalises and calms acid stomach. Spectrumzyme, a digestive enzyme with main meals. BC

READING

The Food Combiners Meal Planner by Kathryn Marsden. £4-99. Thorsons. A valuable handbook about acid and alkaline foods.

HINTS

Stress increases stomach acid, so learn how to relax by joining a local yoga class. Take regular exercise in the fresh air to aid digestion, but not immediately after eating. Ensure meal times are as stress-free and unhurried as possible. If you are upset, exhausted, or in a rush, don't eat a large meal as the digestive system shuts down when under stress. Eat small amounts frequently, avoid drinking with meals as this dilutes digestive secretions which can increase indigestion. Chew all food thoroughly.

ACNE

This chronic skin condition can be triggered by hormones, the Pill, stress or dietary changes and is very common in adolescence. The key to controlling acne is a cleansing diet.

DIET
Try eating only fruit and vegetables accompanied by lots of mineral water for three days; then maintain a healthy diet that includes wholemeal bread, rice, grains and pulses. Above all, avoid red meat and greasy take-away meals which are high in saturated fats, and cut down on sugar, for at least six weeks.

SUPPLEMENTS
15,000iu of Beta Carotene daily to support the skin plus 3 grams of vitamin C.
Zinc is vital as it aids renewal of skin cells. Take Zinc Picolinate 30-60mg daily for six weeks.
Evening Primrose Oil capsules 2 grams daily to help regulate skin hormones.
Take a once a day multi-vitamin which includes minerals. **FSC**

Greenfood supplements such as Green Barley, Chlorella, Blue Green Algae and Spirulina all act as cleansers and help to re-alkalise the system. Available from good health stores.
If you have been on long term antibiotics make sure you take 2 Acidophilus capsules daily to replace the good bacteria in the gut.
Echinacea, the herb has a calming effect on the skin. 2 capsules daily. Made by Solgar, at all good health shops.

READING
Superskin by Kathryn Marsden. £6-99. Thorsons.

HINTS
Chromium is helpful if you have sugar cravings, and is available from most health food shops. If the acne is related to your monthly cycle, add Vitamin B6 to your daily supplements.
The Sher System is a skin regime especially formulated for problem skin and further details can be obtained from The Sher System, 30 New Bond Street, London W1Y 9HD or call 0171-499 4022.
Get plenty of exercise in the fresh air which encourages free flow of the sebum. Many readers have benefited from taking Aloe Vera juice internally and by using the gel externally.

AGEING
Ageing is a natural process, but it is also a state of mind. There is an old adage, you are as old as you feel, which is very true. A positive mental outlook along with a healthy diet is vital if you want to stay happy and healthy. People who are always miserable and negative age faster than happy, relaxed people. As we breathe we generate free radicals which cause ageing. They are also produced when anything is burnt, like cigarettes, toast, fried food, car exhausts and pollution. Free radicals are the primary cause of ageing. While you can't completely avoid them you can protect yourself by taking antioxidant nutrients which render the free radicals harmless. The most important antioxidants are beta carotene, vitamin C, A, E, zinc and selenium. GLA (Gamma Linolenic Acid), an essential fatty acid which is also vital to help keep skin young.

DIET
A healthy diet can slow the ageing process, maintain skin suppleness and decrease spots. There is no point in taking vitamins and supplements for ageing if your diet is unhealthy. Drink at least 1 litre of filtered or bottled water daily. Eat plenty of brown rice, brown bread, lentils, beans, organic vegetables, fruit, nuts and seeds. Avoid sugar, white bread, cakes and biscuits, which have no nutritional value. Avoid saturated fats (found in red meat

and dairy produce) and all junk foods which block the pores and cause ageing. Avoid cigarettes, alcohol, tea and coffee which dehydrate the body. (See also General Health Hints.)

SUPPLEMENTS

Women: Vitamin C as Magnesium Ascorbate 500mg x 3, and one B Complex with enzymes daily. Both essential for the nervous system, skin, nails and hair.

BioGuard Forte one daily which contains beta carotene, vitamin E, selenium and a new high potency antioxidant containing lycopene. All vital to aid prevention of breast, lung and endometrial cancers, and keep you looking healthier.

Zinc Ascorbate one daily to support the immune system.

Women over 40 should also take one Oxidant daily to protect against free radical damage, plus two Femforte, a multi vitamin especially for women.

Co-enzyme Q10 aids energy production, helps protect the heart and aids circulation. CoQ10 Plus, also contains flax seed oil an essential fatty acid which protects the skin and supports the immune system. BC

Men: Vitamin C at least one gram daily plus Zinc Ascorbate to help protect prostate and sperm count. Plus BioGuard Forte one daily along with 300iu of vitamin E to help protect the heart. BC

READING

Ageless Body, Timeless Mind by Deepak Chopra. £7-99. Rider Press.

Optimum Nutrition by Patrick Holford £5.95 ION Press, to order 0181 877 9993.

The New Joy of Beauty by Leslie Kenton. £8-99. Vermilion.

The New Super Nutrition by Richard Passwater £5.99 Pocket Books, to order 0171 436 5122.

HINTS

Stress lowers the immune system and is highly ageing. Make sure that you take plenty of exercise to keep stress to a minimum. There is now a new laser therapy which can remove lines and age spots.

For further details contact Laser Care, 1 Park View, Harrogate, North Yorkshire HG1 5LY Tel 01423 563827.

ALCOHOL CONSUMPTION

For biological reasons, due to their higher percentage of body fat, women tend to become intoxicated sooner than their male counterparts. It is a myth that drinking lots of coffee will help you to sober up or relieve a hangover. Coffee, like alcohol, dehydrates the body and speeds up the rate at which alcohol is absorbed into the blood stream which can actually make you feel more drunk. It helps to drink a large glass of mineral water or juice between alcoholic drinks. Alcohol depletes the body of vital nutrients like vitamin C and B, especially folic acid and vitamin B1.

DIET
Fresh vegetable juice, especially beetroot, is very cleansing for the liver. Fresh raw vegetables, especially broccoli, cabbage, cauliflower and artichokes contain chemicals which help the liver detoxify more efficiently.

SUPPLEMENTS
Alcohol must first be processed by the liver, so take a daily supplement like Nature's Plus Liv R Actin, made from the herb Milk Thistle which is known to help with liver function and cleansing.
Super C Complex plus One Mega Multi daily which is high in B vitamins, along with Natural Flow's Multi-Mineral, which speeds elimination of alcohol from the body. LGF

HINTS
Dandelion Tea is excellent for cleansing the liver and kidneys. If you are concerned about the amount you, or a member of your family, are drinking call Drinkline, a national alcohol Helpline, on 0345 320202 or 0171-332 0202 in London; or their 24hr recorded information service on 0500 801802. All calls are treated in the strictest confidence and Drinkline provides a full support service for people with drink problems as well as their families.

ALLERGIC RHINITIS

Symptoms include a runny nose, congestion, and occasionally sore eyes. Food allergies are often linked with this problem, but an overly restrictive diet can be harmful because too many essential nutrients are removed from every day eating. It can be induced by inhalation of perfume, paint fumes or pollen, also by allergic reactions to animal fur and sudden temperature changes.

DIET
This problem is often associated with an allergy to cow's milk, chocolate, orange juice or wheat. Keep a food diary and make a note of what you have eaten when a bad attack strikes. If you find cow's milk and produce is your problem switch to soya milk or rice milk which are non dairy, low fat and sugar free.

SUPPLEMENTS
Acidophilus to maintain the good bacteria in the gut.
Anti-fungal supplements like echinacea and garlic help build resistance. Super Horseradish and Garlic should help alleviate symptoms during an attack, as will Chloride Compound.
Take 3 grams of Bio C with Bioflavonoids daily, which have a natural anti-histamine effect.
Digestive Enzymes can help ensure proper digestion of foods as inadequate digestion can lead to allergic reactions.
One high potency Multi-vitamin/mineral plus Magnesium and Zinc daily. BLK

READING
Not all in the Mind by Dr Richard Mackarness. £7.99. Thorsons.
The Allergy Survival Guide by Jane Houtton. £10-99. Vermillion.

HINTS
A kinesiologist should determine the cause of your allergy. See index for details of how to find your nearest practitioner. Try New Era Tissue Salts for Allergic Rhinitis from any good pharmacy.

ALLERGIES

There are now over 3,500 food additives in use and an average person ingests 4.5kg of these a year, ten times the amount we ate thirty years ago. A further 3,000 chemicals such as lead and cadmium are in our polluted air. We were not designed to ingest so many chemicals; and for those who suffer allergies, the body is simply saying that it has had enough. We also inhale toxins like paint fumes, hair sprays, deodorants, fly sprays, and perfumes. If you are suffering from any kind of allergy, contact a company called Allergy Care. They provide literature on the subject and give allergy tests, as well as publishing an individual computerised cook book and offering a full mail order food service. Contact them on Allergy Care, Pollards Yard, Wood Street. Taunton. Somerset. TA1 1UP. Tel: 01823 325023.

DIET

Allergies often occur because of bad digestion and when the system is not receiving all the nutrition it needs. This can be due to low stomach acid. Many allergies have their basis in a 'leaky gut' where undigested proteins leak through the gut wall creating a typical allergic response. A natural wholefood diet is likely to be beneficial, and avoid any foods to which you know you are allergic. The commonest allergens are eggs, wheat, yeast dairy produce and oranges. It is often foods that you crave the most that are causing the problem! Most habits and cravings take at least a month to break so be patient with yourself.

SUPPLEMENTS

Histazyme. A natural anti-histamine with vitamin C.
Hepaguard. To help cleanse the liver.
Bio-Acidophilus to replace the good bacteria in the gut.
High Potency Multi-vitamin with extra Vitamin C.
Vitamin E at least 200iu daily, a natural anti-inflammatory. BC

READING

The Allergy Survival Guide by Jane Houtton. £10-99. Vermillion.
Not All In The Mind by Dr Richard Mackarness. £7-99 Thorsons.
Allergy Care Update by Allergy Care. Tel: 01823 325023.

HINTS

Higher Nature now have an allergy test which is 95% accurate, but it is expensive at £295. For details call 01435 882880
See a Kinesiologist who can test for allergens. See index for further details.
Medivac Vacuum Cleaner is an excellent effective high powered vacuum which does not give out dust in its exhaust. Further details available on 01625 539401.

ALZHEIMER'S DISEASE

A progressive, degenerative disease that attacks the brain, resulting in memory loss and decreased intellectual functioning. Many alternative doctors and practitioners now believe that up to 40% of patients are misdiagnosed. According to Dr Abram Hoffer, a pioneer of nutritional medicine in America, "It has come to the point that anyone over 65 with the slightest memory loss is in danger of being labelled with Alzheimer's."

SUPPLEMENTS

In Japan studies showed that a daily supplement of Co-enzyme Q10, vitamin B6 and iron compounds returned some patients to normal functioning. Other studies listed benefits from evening primrose oil to zinc and selenium.

Deficiency in the vital nutrient Acetylcholine results in poor memory, lethargy, decreased dreaming and a dry mouth. Take lecithin granules daily on your cereal, but make sure the product you buy contains more than 30% of phosphatidyl choline. Also take a supplement called Brain Food which contains all the nutrients necessary to increase Acetylcholine levels, three daily. For details call Higher Nature 01435 882880. Studies have shown that a daily intake of Ginkgo Biloba and Phosphatidylserine improves micro circulation, memory and behaviour. Also take an antioxidant complex, plus 200iu of vitamin E daily to improve oxygen supply to the brain. For details call 0121-433 3727.

READING

Coping With Alzheimer's - A Care Givers Emotional Survival Guide by Rose Oliver and Frances Bock. £8.99. Wilshire Books.

Alzheimer's and Other Confusional States by Dr Gerry Bennett. £5.99. Optima.

Alzheimer's - A Practical Guide For Carers To Help You Through The Day by Frena Gray-Davidson. £8.99. Piatkus Books.

Volume 5, no 12 of What Doctors Don't Tell You. £2.90. See index for further details.

HINTS

Certain prescription drugs are known to cause side effects which appear as senile dementia. Anyone who feels that they may have the onset of dementia should immediately see a qualified doctor who is also a nutritionist. See index. Low blood sugar can also cause dementia type symptoms, (see Low Blood Sugar). In certain cases, having amalgam fillings removed has assisted with the recovery of some faculties, (see Mercury Fillings). Aluminium has been linked to Alzheimers, therefore avoid aluminium cooking utensils and pans, any food stored in aluminium containers, and antacids which contain aluminium. Some readers report that homeopathy has improved their condition. Make sure you see a homeopath who is also a qualified doctor. See index for further details.

ANGINA

Angina Pectoris is caused by lack of oxygen reaching the heart muscle usually brought on by exertion. Typical symptoms include a constricting pain in the centre of the chest which may spread to the neck and the jaw, or to the shoulders down one or both arms to the hand. It is sometimes accompanied by breathlessness, faintness, sweating, nausea or breathing problems.

DIET

If angina has been diagnosed, start eating a healthier diet. Avoid eating junk foods like take away burgers, which contain high levels of salt and sugar; raising blood pressure and bringing on an attack of angina. Eat plenty of oily fish like mackerel, herrings and salmon, which contain omega 3 oils known to protect the heart. Use extra virgin olive oil which is the highest quality mono-unsaturated fat, instead of saturated animal fats. Never fry your food; steam, boil, roast or grill. Eat plenty of fresh fruit, vegetables and whole grains like brown rice and pulses. Garlic is known to thin the blood, so use plenty in cooking and eat it raw whenever possible.

SUPPLEMENTS
Bio-Magnesium to help regulate heart beat.
BioGuard Forte containing Beta Carotene, vitamin E and selenium, all vital nutrients to assist the heart muscle and aid circulation.
Ginkgo Plus containing bilberry and potassium ascorbate to strengthen capillaries and improve circulation. BC
Co-enzyme Q10 is known to protect the heart, a particularly good formula is Bio Quinone Q10 by Pharma Nord, for details call 0800 591 756. If you are not on blood thinning drugs, take a garlic capsule regularly.

READING
The Natural Way With Heart Disease by Richard Thomas. £3-99. Element Books.
Coping With Angina by Louise M Wallace. £7-99. Thorsons.
Super Nutrition for a Healthy Heart by Patrick Holford £2.50 ION Press.

HINTS
Lose weight sensibly if obese and stop smoking. With your doctor's permission, embark on a programme of gentle exercise. Start by walking for fifteen minutes daily, gradually building to thirty minutes. Join a yoga class, an excellent form of relaxation which reduces stress and teaches you how to breathe properly.

Linus Pauling's New Theory of Heart Disease video. £9.95 from The Institute of Optimum Nutrition Tel 0181 877 9993. Explains how people have been helped by Mega Doses of Vitamin C and Lysine.

ANTIBIOTICS (See also Candida)

Long term use of antibiotics has a negative affect on the body by destroying the good bacteria in the gut along with the undesirable bacteria which can cause the infections. Bacteria develop an immunity to antibiotics over time, creating new resistant strains of bacteria which attack the immune system. Consistent courses of antibiotics suppress the immune system and allow fungal infections to flourish in the body. There are specific supplements which will help to protect your immune system.

DIET

Keep your diet really clean for a few weeks. Eat lots of wholegrains, like brown rice, porridge, along with pulses, fresh fruit and plenty of raw or steamed vegetables, preferably organic as they have less additives and pesticides. No red meat, but organic free range poultry is permissible as it is unlikely to contain the antibiotic residues commonly found in non-organic sources of meat and poultry.

SUPPLEMENTS

If you have been taking antibiotics in the long term then take Acidophilus daily on an empty stomach to replace the friendly bacteria in the gut which helps restore the immune and digestive systems.

You also need to replace the B vitamins in the body especially Biotin with a B Complex.

Try a new natural alternative to antibiotics called Citricidal made from grapefruit seeds which kills the bad bacteria without harming the body's natural balance. A few drops in juice daily will help fight an infection. For details call 01435 882880.

READING

Superbug. Nature's Revenge by Geoffrey Cannon. £15-99. Virgin Books.

HINTS

A naturopath or nutritionist will be able to help restore your immune system. See index for further details.

Aphrodisiacs (MALE)

DIET
Make sure your diet is high in vegetables and fruit and low in animal fat and salt. Red meat should be replaced by free range chicken and fish. Caffeine and alcohol intake should be limited as excessive consumption can have an adverse effect on libido. Smoking can also affect libido and potency - so give up!

SUPPLEMENTS
There is a supplement made especially for men called Virilactin which includes vitamins like B and E and the mineral zinc which are vital for male glandular activity. Also extracts of oysters, a natural source of zinc, and herbs like Kava Kava, Dong Quai and Spanish Saffron, all recognised for their aphrodisiac qualities. LGF
Formula 600 for men ensures a healthier prostate and contains aphrodisiac herbs. FSC

READING
Optimum Nutrition by Patrick Holford £5.95 ION Press.
The Complete Book of Men's Health by Dr Sara Brewer. £9.99. Thorsons.

HINTS
Eat plenty of pumpkin seeds which are high in zinc, essential for a healthy libido. Make sure you get plenty of exercise and fresh air to aid relaxation. By constant worrying about lack of sex drive, you often make the situation worse. Recent studies show that a lack of vitamin C, E, A, B and zinc can cause a lowered sperm count and lack of sex drive. Anyone taking regular anti-depressants or sleeping pills will be lacking in these supplements. If the condition continues or you are worried about infertility as well as impotency see a doctor who is also a nutritionist. See index for further details.

ARTHRITIS

A degenerative condition of the joints. The two most common being Osteo and Rheumatoid Arthritis. Osteo arthritis is caused when cartilage inside the joints wears away and can result from an injury. Rheumatoid arthritis is a chronic inflammatory condition primarily affecting the joints but can also affect the skin, lymph nodes, heart, lungs, blood and nervous systems. One in six people are affected including 80% over the age of 70.

DIET

Some people who have written to me about this complaint are often overweight and their diet is far too high in acid forming foods. Throughout this book, this theme appears many times; and to my mind it is one of the root causes of many of our degenerative diseases. Avoid all junk and take-away foods like hamburgers and shop bought cakes as they are high in salt and sugar. Tea, coffee, alcohol, colas, sugary drinks, red meat, sausages, refined white flour products; bread, cakes and biscuits are all acid forming. Don't fry food. Eat plenty of fresh fruit salad, but avoid oranges, rhubarb and plums which are acidic. Include lots of green vegetables especially cabbage, broccoli and kale in your daily diet. Eat plenty of oily fish like salmon and mackerel, and if you must eat meat only choose free range poultry. Use extra virgin olive oil for cooking and salad dressings. Include linseeds in your diet every day, I have found that Linusit Gold is one of the better brands, from all health stores. If you have a juicer, try the following daily: carrot, celery, cabbage and a tiny piece of chopped fresh root ginger which is highly anti-inflammatory. Make your own vegetable mix daily, but drink it straight from the juicer while the enzymes and vitamins are 'alive'.

Arthritis can be aggravated by food allergies and many people should avoid the most common culprits which are found in the nightshade family; tomatoes, potatoes, red and green peppers, and aubergines. Fifty per cent of arthritis sufferers react to wheat or dairy produce.

SUPPLEMENTS

Ligazyme, a natural anti-inflammatory supplement plus Colleginase with each meal to support connective tissue and aid healing. Bio-Acidophilus on an empty stomach to replace good bacteria in the gut and aid digestion. BC
Joint Nutritional Complex containing Shark Cartilage, Glucosamine, DLPA and Vitamin B5, has proven useful for arthritis, especially osteo. LGF
Glucosamine Sulphate has proved helpful in chronic arthritis, particularly where mobility is impaired. Cat's Claw is a herb that helps to alkalise the system and is highly anti-inflamatory. Take a concentrated fish oil like Super EPA daily. Both Cat's Claw and EPA are made by Solgar. NC

HINTS

Many readers have accredited relief to the following items:

A preparation of fresh Royal Jelly made with Ginseng and Echinacea, an immune system booster and natural antibiotic, is helpful for arthritis. For further details send a large SAE to: Irene Stein, 67c Camlet Way, Hadley Wood, Hertfordshire EN4 0NL.

Green Barley Plus and SeaCare, which alkalise the system. For details call 0181 504 2755, or send an SAE to Nature's Wealth, 40 Forrest Way, Woodford Wells, Essex IG9 0QS.

Wearing magnets has given relief from the pain. For details of the magnetic aids send an SAE to Acar-Sud, Westfield House, Hampton Court Road, East Molesey, Surrey KT8 9BX. Tel. 0181 977 1699.

Homeopathic remedies, acupuncture, Chinese herbs, taking stabilised aloe vera juice or by seeing a qualified nutritionist. See index for further details.

For help, ideas and counselling on arthritis call: Arthritis Care on their Freephone Helpline between 12 to 4pm Monday to Friday 0800 289170.
Arthritic Association call 0171 491 0233. This charity provides very good dietary advice - yearly membership costs £6.

READING
Say No to Arthritis by Patrick Holford. £5.95. ION Press.
Arthritis by Stephen Terrass. £4.99. Thorsons.
Exercise Beats Arthritis by Valerie Sayce. £9.99. Thorsons.
The Natural Way With Arthritis and Rheumatism by Pat Young. £3.99. Element Books.

ASTHMA (See also Allergies)

This is a condition in which breathing is made difficult by muscle spasms and increased mucus in the lining of the bronchial tubes. Check to see if you are allergic to environmental allergens such as pet hairs, dust, feathers, paints, perfume, pollen or the house dust mite. To check for food and environmental allergens see a kinesiologist to determine what foods and household items you need to avoid. Stay away from cigarette smoke at all times. According to The Lancet, low magnesium levels have been found in many patients suffering asthma and chronic airway diseases. Most asthma drugs deplete magnesium levels.

DIET
Avoid mucous forming foods like cow's milk, bread, cakes, cheese, chocolate and biscuits. Reduce intake of salt, any junk foods, fizzy drinks, sugar, nuts and seafood. Avoid foods and drinks that have been preserved with sulphur, such as dried fruits, wines, beers and commercially produced salads. Vitally important in the control of asthma is the elimination of all food additives (See Allergies). Artificial dyes and preservatives can often trigger an attack. Diet should be rich in dark green leaf and orange vegetables, garlic, onions, fresh salmon, mackerel, sardines and extra virgin olive oil. If you have a juicer, try carrot and radish juice daily. If eating margarines instead of butter, opt for those which specifically avoid inclusion of trans-fatty acids like Vitaquell and SuperSpread. Also include linseeds, linseed oil and pumpkin seeds in the diet. A vegan diet has been found helpful when followed for at least twelve months.

SUPPLEMENTS
Natural Flow's Super C Complex for a natural anti-histamine effect.
Nature's Plus Magnesium 200mg daily. Antoxymega is a one-a-day
advanced Antioxidant formula with Bioflavonoids. LGF
To help heal a leaky gut which often contributes to asthma also
take Magnesium Ascorbate plus NAG daily. (N. Acetyl
Glucosamine), helps to heal tissue. For details call 0121 433 3727.

READING
New Self Help For Asthma by Leon Chaitow. £2.99. Thorsons.
The Asthma Action Plan by John Chapman. £5.99. Thorsons.
The Natural Way With Asthma by Roy Ridgeway. £3.99.
Element Books.

HINTS
Colonic Irrigation has proved helpful for many sufferers.
Readers have found relief from asthma by seeing homeopathic
doctors or a nutritionist. See index for further details. Honeywell
make a room air filter called Enviracare which removes all known
allergens. For details call Essential Systems on 01344 874 573.
Asthma Helpline 0345 010203
National Asthma Campaign Information packs are available by
dialling 0891 441188.

ATHLETE'S FOOT
A chronic fungal infection of the superficial skin of the foot,
especially between the toes and on the soles. Symptoms include
peeling of the skin, soreness, itching and cracked and softened
skin. The condition is easily transmitted in public places where
people walk barefoot. All fungal infections thrive in a moist
atmosphere so wear natural fibres that allow your feet to breathe,
dry in between your toes thoroughly after washing and avoid
wearing tight fitting shoes. Persistent athlete's foot is often
associated with an overgrowth of Candida in the gut, see Candida.

DIET
Avoid any foods that contain sugar. Try Pau D'arco tea from your health shop. Keep your diet really clean and eat lots of wholegrains, like brown rice along with pulses, fresh fruit and plenty of raw or steamed vegetables. See General Health Hints.

SUPPLEMENTS
Tea Tree Oil is a powerful anti-fungal agent. Add a few drops to your bath water or foot bath and soak your feet for 10 minutes before bed each night.
Acidophilus daily on an empty stomach, to restore healthy bacteria in the gut which is essential in fighting fungal infections.
Dab the affected areas with Kyolic Liquid Garlic and take the odourless tablets internally. Q
Cervagen cream can be applied to the affected area. BC

BACK PAIN

Back pain accounts for the loss of twenty million working days each year and two thirds of all back sufferers are under the age of 40. Back pain is often due to poor posture or by lifting incorrectly. It can also be caused by a kidney or lung infection like pleurisy. If back pain does not settle within a few days or if you are in severe pain, see your doctor. Many GP's refer their patients to a good chiropractor or osteopath. If you wear a corset you often encourage the muscles to atrophy, whereas certain sports like swimming can strengthen back muscles.

DIET
Avoid smoking which reduces oxygen supply to muscles including the back. Stick to a low fat good wholefood diet and drink plenty of filtered water. See General Health Hints.

SUPPLEMENTS
Glucosamine Sulphate is a supplement which helps to restore the thick, gelatinous nature of the fluids and tissues around the joints and in-between the vertebrae. Its effectiveness in relieving back pain is enhanced if taken with a good Antioxidant formula, such as Solgar's Advanced Antioxidant Complex capsules. NC

Magnesium Malate has proved useful for pain relief. Also Ligazyme - developed by a chiropractor to help with skeletal problems. Take 2 Mega GLA daily, an essential fatty acid known to have an anti-inflamatory effect. BC

READING
The Natural Way With Back Pain by Helena Bridge. £3.99. Element Books.
Treat Your Own Back by Robin McKenzie. £7.99. To order call ProCare Medipost Ltd on 0161-678 0233

HINTS
Empulse is a pulsed electromagnetic treatment, the setting of which is governed by an analysis of the brain's electrical activity. It is a non-invasive, non-drug based treatment. Further details are available from: MDI Ltd, 17 Owen Road, Diss, Norfolk IP22 3ER or call 01379 644234
A helpful video is Your Back, An Owners Guide To Its Care and Maintenance by Professor Diane Newham, England's first Professor of Physiotherapy. £10.99 plus p&p from Eye Eye Ltd on 0171-700 3555. This one hour video will teach you about back care and maintenance, plus emergency exercise which can be used when you are in pain.
For a large information pack, send £2 to the Back Pain Association, 16 Elm Tree Road, Teddington, Middlesex TW11 8ST.

BAD BREATH
(see Halitosis)

BEREAVEMENT
Because I have written quite regularly about life after death, I have received many letters from people who have lost a loved one. Their desolation and feelings of isolation are heartbreaking. I have a strong belief in life after death, which definitely has nothing to do with the occult or religion. After my mother died I derived great comfort from imagining her near me and by talking to her.

It is important for you to be able to share your feelings with someone who has gone through a similar experience. In death we all wish there were things we had said and done; regrets, guilt and the seemingly endless emotion of desperately wanting to see that loved one again. It is normal to grieve for a few months, but as time passes the hurt should lessen a little. Crying lets out the emotion as tears shed in trauma contain a high level of stress chemicals , so a good cry really can bring relief. Professional counselling is invaluable if you find you cannot let go and the depression does not lift.

Also it is easy to forget to eat properly under such painful conditions, but remember that by making an effort to look after yourself with a balanced diet and exercise, this will help you to cope. Try a Bach Rescue Remedy, available from good health stores.

READING
A Time to Grieve by Carol Staudacher. £9.99. Souvenir Press.
Testimony of Light by Helen Graves. £5.95. Published by
Neville Spearman to order call Watkins Books on 0171 836 2182.
Embraced by the Light by Betty J Eadie. £4.99. Aquarian Press.

HINTS
Cruse Bereavement Care, a charity founded in 1959 which has 180 branches in the UK. For further information write to Cruse Bereavement Care, 126 Sheen Road, Richmond, Surrey, TW9 1UR or call 0181-940 4818.

Compassionate Friends is a nationwide organisation of bereaved parents offering friendship and understanding. Quarterly Newsletter, Postal Library and a range of leaflets. Befriending rather than counselling. For further information contact. The Compassionate Friends, 53 North Street, Bristol BS3 1EN Helpline 01179 539639.

BLADDER (see Cystitis, Incontinence, Prostate)

BLEEDING GUMS

The bleeding can be caused by excessively vigorous brushing, or a reaction to certain toothpastes and strong mouthwashes as well as by gum infections. Smoking is a factor in gum disease because tobacco smoke is highly toxic and stimulates the build up of plaque. Make sure you see an oral hygienist and a dentist at least twice annually for a thorough clean and check up.

DIET
Bacteria thrive on sugar and starch, so keep your diet as clean as possible by avoiding all junk foods. Eat plenty of green vegetables, fruit and wholegrains. (See General Health Hints).

SUPPLEMENTS
Vitamin C Complex with Bioflavonoids. Co-enzyme Q10, which aids healing of the gums plus Silica to increase strength of connective tissue and reduce bleeding.

HINTS
Practise good daily dental hygiene by using a floss and a natural mouthwash like Paracidin (2oz diluted in warm water, do not swallow). BC
Clean teeth and gums daily with a water pick, adding a few drops of Tea Tree Oil and one drop of Clove Oil, which is an excellent antiseptic, to the warm water. Chewing sugar free gum after a meal helps release saliva, which is alkaline and counteracts the gum/tooth damaging acids in foods.Use a good herbal toothpaste like Sarakan or Blackmores.

BLEPHARITIS

A condition where calcium deposits lodge under the eyelids causing inflammation.

DIET

Eat more green vegetables and citrus fruits. Avoid red meats and cheese, spinach, chocolate, sugar and animal fats. Bioflavonoid rich foods like bilberries, blueberries, cherries are known to soothe the eyes.

SUPPLEMENTS

Mega GLA daily - an essential fatty acid which is anti-inflamatory.
Procydin, contains bilberry and blackberry extracts which are high in bioflavonoids known to support delicate eye tissue.
Bio Guard containing Beta Carotene, selenium and vitamin E one daily.
Bio-Magnesium helps keep calcium in suspension which may stop the deposits forming. BC

A compress made with cucumber helps to reduce inflammation. Drink Rose Hip Tea daily which contains bioflavonoids and vitamin C. Natural Flow Eyebright and Ocutrien, a comprehensive eye nutrition formula by ophthalmic nutritionist Dr Stanley Evans. Se-power a selenium/vitamin/herbal formula for eye health. LGF

HINTS

Mix one teaspoonful of bicarbonate of soda with one pint of boiled water. Allow to cool, then apply to the blisters inside your eyelid with a cotton bud.

BODY ODOUR

Body odour can be aggravated by anxiety which produces sweating, or by an unhealthy or over spicy diet. Daily bathing or showering is essential, especially after exercise along with a regular change of underclothes.

DIET
Eat a balanced wholefood diet high in fruits and vegetables and low in animal fats and red meats which can putrify in the gut causing odour. See General Health Hints.

SUPPLEMENTS
Incomplete breakdown of foods can cause body odour, therefore Digestive Enzymes with main meals can be helpful, together with Acidophilus.
Deficiency of Zinc is sometimes related to excessive perspiration so try taking a high potency multi-vitamin to support the whole system such as Mega-Multi and Natural Flows Multi-Mineral. LGF
Green food supplements such as Green Magna and Chlorella contain high levels of Chlorophyll which counteracts odour and bacteria.

HINTS
If persistent body odour is present this could indicate liver dysfunction, diabetes, digestive problems and/or yeast infections, which should be investigated further therefore see a doctor who is also a nutritiionist. See index for details.
PitRok - a natural odourless mineral salt deodorant which prevents bacterial growth without the use of harsh chemicals or aluminium. Just wet the crystal and glide it over the skin. Available from most health food shops. Or call PitRok on 0181-563 1120.

BOILS

A boil is an acute bacterial infection of hair follicles with surrounding inflammation. Often associated with stress and worry which lowers the immune system. Recurrent boils can also stem from a poor diet or be an early sign of diabetes. Ask your GP for a thorough check up. Clean up your diet, and eat foods that will boost the immune system.

DIET

Avoid all red meat which can putrify in the gut. Eat plenty of green and yellow vegetables along with apples, pears, bananas and grapes whilst avoiding strawberries, pineapples and oranges. Drink plenty of water to avoid becoming constipated. Reduce tea, coffee, sugary drinks, take-away foods and all alcohol intake. See General Health Hints.

SUPPLEMENTS

Garlic is an effective antiseptic and helps to detoxify the body therefore eat the raw herb daily or take an odour free garlic tablet like Kwai daily with your main meal.

Take supplements to help cleanse the liver such as Vitamin C, Acidophilus, Vitamin E, Zinc Ascorbate and Sea Plasma. BC

Tea Tree Oil, a natural antiseptic, is excellent for boils and can be applied neat if required, available from good health food shops.

READING

Superskin by Kathryn Marsden. £6.99. Thorsons.

HINTS

Make sure you get plenty of exercise in the fresh air and always wash after exercise. Saunas may be beneficial to clear blocked pores and drain toxins from the body.

Colonic irrigation therapy is a thorough but gentle way to cleanse the bowel and rid the body of toxins. See index for further details.

BRAIN (see also Memory)

Many aspects of brain function remain a mystery to us, but what we do know is that the brain responds to use and need not degenerate over time. It is said to be the most self-rejuvenating organ in the body provided it is kept in use! Studies have shown that the brain is made entirely out of food molecules, and that sixty percent of all nutrients passed from the mother to her unborn baby are used by the brain for it's development. In an adult 30% of all energy derived from food is used by the brain. Bad nutrition has been identified with hyperactivity, learning difficulties, delinquent behaviour, depression, anxiety, schizophrenia, insomnia, memory loss and anorexia; in fact, almost every known mental health problem. The brain consumes as much as 40% of the oxygen we breathe. Therefore exercise which encourages a higher intake of oxygen and increases circulation is vital to brain function.

For anyone who is concerned about mental illness read Mental Illness - Not All In The Mind, a booklet by Patrick Holford. £1.25. Available from the Institute for Optimum Nutrition, Blades Court, Deodar Road, London SW15 2NU.

For supplements to help brain function- See under Memory.

BREAST PAIN (see also Cancer of the Breast)

Breast pain or mastalgia can be a cyclical phenomenon in women often occurring pre-menstrually. It is often caused by poor lymphatic drainage in the fatty tissue under the arms. Professional manual lymphatic drainage is a gentle massage technique known to improve drainage of toxins from the area, and reducing swelling and pain. Breast discomfort in the first three months of pregnancy is usual. If the pain in the breast is present for most of the month, or if it is severe, then a doctor should be consulted. Other breast problems include breast lumps which should immediately be reported to a doctor.

DIET

To avoid water retention cut down on salt, reduce alcohol and coffee as well as saturated fat intake. Eating plenty of fresh fruits, vegetables, low fat protein and whole grains will aid de-toxification. Coffee is particularly associated with breast pain. Regularly including soya products and vegetables such as cabbage, broccoli and cauliflower have a hormone modulating effect. Eat vegetables raw for maximum effect. Kombu Seaweed contains iodine known to relieve mastitis type breast pain or take Kelp.

SUPPLEMENTS

Vitamin B6 200-400mg daily, plus a multi-vitamin for women like Femforte. BC

Take 1 garlic tablet for cleansing plus 300iu of vitamin E daily. Efamol Evening Primrose Oil at least 2 capsules daily.

Red Clover tea is an excellent blood cleanser, as are Blue Flag Root Tablets by Gerard House available from all good health shops.

If after three months there is no improvement, see a qualified doctor who is also a nutritionist. See index for details.

READING

Your Breasts. What Every Woman Needs To Know by Brian Butler. £9.95 Task Books, PO Box 359a, Surbiton, Surrey. KT5 8YP Call 0181 399 3215.

HINTS

Regular exercise improves circulation and aids drainage of the lymph system. Rebounders (mini trampolines) are wonderful for this problem as is any vigorous exercise such as fast walking, swimming or dancing.

Have a manual lymphatic drainage (MLD) massage, a gentle but effective way to drain the lymph nodes thereby reducing pain and tenderness. See index for details.

BRUISING

A discoloration seen through the skin after the breaking of blood vessels, usually after trauma or injury.

Arnica is a homeopathic remedy which aids healing of internal and external bruising and is especially good for helping with the shock to ones system after any surgery. It aids recovery from mental and physical shock. When I recently had surgery on my teeth which had previously caused a huge amount of swelling, I took Arnica tablets under my tongue twice before the operation and every two hours for two days post operatively and had virtually no swelling! You can also apply Arnica cream topically and iced Witch Hazel compresses.

DIET
Wholefood diet which includes plenty of salads, fresh vegetables and fruits. To avoid bruising stop taking aspirin, excessive tea, coffee and alcohol before surgery.

SUPPLEMENTS
Vitamin C Complex which includes bioflavonoids to help strengthen capillaries. Bromelain is an anti-inflammatory flavonoid derived from pineapple, 500mg x 3 times daily on an empty stomach if you have bad bruising.
A high potency multi-vitamin like Green Multi daily. FSC
READING
Arnica The Wonder Herb by Phyllis Speight. £3.75. From Nelsons Mail Order, 73 Duke Street, London W1 or call 0171-495 2404.

CANCER

In many cases, the exact cause of cancers are not known. There is however, a very strong relationship between smoking and lung cancer. Melanoma of the skin and excessive exposure to sunshine. It is possible that there are certain chemicals in the diet that may well be shown to be responsible for certain tumours. Some virus infections are also associated with cancer. From all the hundreds of cancer patients I have met and interviewed, it seems to me that alternative and orthodox treatments can work really well side by side to help destroy many cancers which were previously thought incurable.

The Alternative Anti Cancer Diet

Avoid fried food. This is the best way to cut down on your exposure to 'free radicals'. These dangerous chemicals are like the nuclear waste of any burning process, in this case oil. Free radicals damage cells and trigger cancer. Boil, steam or bake, eating most of your food raw or lightly cooked. Try 'steam-frying' food using a watered down soya sauce, plus herbs or spices for taste.

Minimise pollution. Anything that is combusted produces free radicals. So the less time you spend exposed to car exhaust and other people's smoke, the better. Barbecued food, burnt food, is also best kept to a minimum.

Eat broccoli, carrots and soya. These three foods have been found to contain anti-cancer chemicals. Soya and broccoli contain substances that counteract hormone excesses associated with breast cancer. Carrots are rich in beta-carotene, high levels of which mean a low risk of cancer. Put two carrots, two heads of broccoli, half a pack of tofu (soya bean curd), a teaspoon of vegetable stock and some water in the blender for a delicious immune boosting soup. Add soya milk if you want it creamy, and spices if you like it hot. Heat and serve.

Eat organic as much as possible. Carrots, lettuce and many other healthy foods are overloaded with pesticides that are associated with an increased risk of cancer. So, whenever possible, eat organic. But, for non-organic vegetables like cabbage or lettuce, throw away the outer leaves. Just one serving of cabbage each week can reduce the risk of colon cancer by 60%.

Eat at least three pieces of fruit a day. Vitamin C and beta-carotene are the most potent anti-cancer nutrients. They are Antioxidants, which protect your body cells from the damage that initiates the development of cancer. Fresh fruit contains lots of vitamin C. Red and orange coloured fruits, such as oranges, apricots or watermelon, are loaded with beta-carotene. Eat fresh fruit as a snack throughout the day.

Eat wholefoods, nuts, beans and seeds. Anything in its whole form, such as oats, brown rice, lentils, almonds or sunflower seeds are high in the essential anti-cancer minerals zinc and selenium. These protect the body from the free radicals that trigger cancer.

Supplement your diet with antioxidant nutrients. Antioxidant nutrients are the most potent anti-cancer agents. Many scientific studies have found low rates of cancer in people who have high levels of antioxidants in their blood. The antioxidant nutrients are primarily vitamin A, beta-carotene, vitamin C, vitamin E, and the minerals zinc and selenium.

Minimise alcohol. Alcohol is a powerful anti-nutrient. In excess, it is associated with an increased risk of cancer. Red wine does contain these antioxidant nutrients, so one glass a day is the recommended maximum. Red grape juice contains the same antioxidants without the alcohol.

READING
Cancer The Positive Approach by Karel Sikora and Hilary Thomas. £8.99. Thorsons.
Cancer and Its Nutritional Therapies by Dr Richard Passwater. £12.50 To order call 0181 877 9993.

HINTS FOR CANCER PATIENTS RECEIVING TREATMENT
If you are already undergoing any type of cancer therapy Dr Rosy Daniel the medical director of the Bristol Cancer Help Centre says that nutrition is vital to help bring up the white blood cell count. She advises patients to eat plenty of organic fresh fruit and vegetables along with whole foods like brown rice and brown bread. All animal fats should be avoided. A daily bottle of Guinness helps to improve blood count as it contains iron and folic acid. She also recommends that cancer patients take a good antioxidant formula which contains vitamin C, Beta Carotene, zinc and selenium. Dr Daniel stresses that fear drains energy levels and advocates any therapy that can reduce anxiety, such as spiritual healing, relaxation exercises, visualisation, acupuncture or homeopathy.

There are many associations which offer help, counselling and advice if you are suffering cancer and need help.

Bristol Cancer Help Centre, Grove House, Cornwallis Grove, Clifton, Bristol BS8 4PG. Patient helpline 01179 743216.

BACUP, 3, Bath Place, Rivington Street, London EC2A 3JR. They offer counselling and advice on cancer and give advice where to find alternative help in your area. Helpline open Monday-Thursday 10am to 7pm. Fridays 10am to 5.30pm. Tel. 0800 181199.

CANCER OF THE BREASTS

Cancer is the leading cause of premature death in women. More than a third of all cancer deaths are diet related. Many scientists now believe there is a link between pesticides like Lindane which we all ingest with meat and vegetables. Most pesticides are fat soluble and therefore end up in the fatty tissue of our breasts. Many nutritional doctors also believe that many women suffering from breast cancer are lacking Beta Carotene. HRT has also been linked to the onset of breast cancer. I personally take a new natural HRT. For details see under Menopause.

DIET

Nature provides natural anti-cancer agents in certain foods, predominantly fruit, vegetables and seeds. These are rich in Beta Carotene, vitamin C, vitamin E and zinc and selenium. The best foods are fresh and colourful. Red/orange foods like carrots or tomatoes are rich in beta carotene, a form of vitamin A. Mauve/blue foods are rich in other antioxidants, as found in berries and beetroot. All fruit contains plenty of vitamin C. Avoid alcohol and if you have been on the birth pill for some time consider an alternative.

Breast cancer and other hormonally related cancers, such as of the uterus, prostate or endometriosis, are associated with excesses of herbicides, pesticides and antibiotics which enter the food chain via animal meats, fruit and vegetables. Therefore reduce meat and cow's milk. Broccoli and soya products such as tofu, which is soya bean curd, contain specific compounds that help to correct hormonal imbalances and are highly protective against breast cancer.

SUPPLEMENTS
A programme that may help prevent breast cancer is; Beta Carotene 25,000iu, Ester Vitamin C at least 3 grams daily, Zinc Picolinate, Selenium, Coenzyme Q10, Kelp, Magnesium Citrate, Vitamin E 200 iu, vitamin D 400 iu, an Advanced Antioxidant Formula and a B complex. All made by Solgar available from good health stores.

READING
Your Breasts. What Every Woman Needs To Know by Brian Butler. £9.95 Task Books, PO Box 359a, Surbiton, Surrey KT5 8YP. Tel: 0181-399 3215.
Breast Cancer, What You Should Know and May Not Be Told About Prevention, Diagnosis and Treatment by Dr Steven Austin and Cathy Hitchcock. £8-99. Prima Press. Call Bookpoint on 01235 400 400.
Cancer and its Nutritional Therapies by Dr Richard Passwater. £12.50 To order call 0181 877 9993.

HINTS
Bristol Cancer Help Centre, Grove House, Cornwallis Grove, Clifton, Bristol BS8 4PG Patient helpline 01179 743216 between 9am - 5pm Monday to Friday.

CANDIDA
Candida Albicans is a yeast which commonly causes superficial infections in the mouth or vagina. Candida in its initial stages is fairly easy to eliminate by keeping to a diet free of yeast products which keeps the bowels clean and helps to prevent the candida spreading. Once the candida goes to the second stage, which is known as Mycelial Fungal Form, it is much harder to treat and far more invasive.

DIET

Keep to a healthy diet. Eat plenty of vegetables, fish and free range poultry and whole grain cereals, whilst avoiding products containing sugar, alcohol and yeast. Buy yeast free breads from your local health store. Also avoid foods like Bovril, Marmite, mushrooms, blue cheese, soy sauce, vinegar and alcohol which are full of yeast. Eat plenty of organic, live, low fat yoghurt. Initially restrict fruit to a minimum because of its natural sugar content.

SUPPLEMENTS

Bio-Acidophilus capsules twice daily to replace the good bacteria in the gut plus garlic to help eliminate the Candida.

Mycopryl, made from time released caprylic acid, to inhibit yeast overgrowth. (Do not take if pregnant or suffering intestinal ulcers).

For more resistant cases, take Candicidin (not if pregnant), a powerful anti-fungal agent which helps rid the entire system of candida two or three times daily. BC

The herb Pau D'arco has anti fungal properties and can be taken daily while the condition lasts. Made by Solgar.

READING

Candida Albicans, A User's Guide To Treatment And Recovery by Gill Jacobs. £7.99. Optima.

Candida Albicans by Shirley Trickett. £7.99. Thorsons.

Could Yeast Be Your Problem by Leon Chaitow. £3.99. To order call 0181 877 9993.

Candida and Thrush, a very useful pamphlet by Dr George Lewith. £2.95 plus p&p from Bio-Med Publications Ltd, 16 Court Oak Grove, Harbourne, Birmingham B32 2HR

The Practical Guide To Candida is a UK directory of practitioners who treat candida naturopathically. £5.75. Green Library, 9 Rickett Street, Fulham, London SW6 1RU.

HINTS

For further help and advice on Candida infections send an SAE and £2 to The Candida Support Group, 10 Burghley Road, London NW5 1UE.

CATARRH

Chronic catarrh problems often stem from a sensitivity to certain foods such as dairy produce and sometimes to carbohydrates like bread, cakes and biscuits which are full of wheat, yeast, gluten and sugar. It can also be related to air-borne allergens such as dust mites. If you have chronic catarrh and are coughing up sputum, see your doctor as you may be suffering from bronchitis.

DIET
By improving your diet and digestion the condition is often alleviated. Keep your diet as clean as possible, eat a little of everything but keep a note when the problem is most severe. Avoid shop bought white bread, cakes, biscuits, sugar based foods and drinks and salt. Stick to a food combining diet for three months. Avoid cow's milk, full fat yoghurts, yeast, sugar, wheat products, oranges and alcohol, full fat cheeses and chocolate. Use soya milk or rice milk which are non-dairy, low fat and sugar free. Drink plenty of filtered water.

SUPPLEMENTS
Muccolyte daily with half a glass of water. Helps to maintain mucus membranes. This may initially make the problem worse but keep going until the course is finished. Vitamin C with Bioflavonoids. BC Garlic tablets like Kwai with your main meal. (Odour Free). The herb Fenugreek is a useful expectorant made in capsule form by Solgar available at any good health store. Also try New Era Tissue Salts for catarrh.

READING
Food Combining in 30 Days by Kathryn Marsden. £5.99. Thorsons.

HINTS
Invest in a humidifier/air filter available from health shops.
See a Kinesiologist to discover which foods are a problem. See index for further details.
Try the new allergy test from Higher Nature, for details call 01435 882880.
Inhale a mixture of cooled boiled water, mixed with a small amount

of olive oil and a pinch of salt to wash out the sinuses. I do this by simply splashing the mixture into the palm of my hand and inhaling it. Not pleasant - but effective!

CHILBLAINS

Chilblains are an inflammation that produce swelling, and may be itchy and painful when the fingers or toes become warm. Chilblains resemble a mild form of frost bite. The answer is to improve your micro circulation.

DIET
Low saturated fat diet, but include a little olive oil and oily fish like salmon and mackerel. Avoid coffee, sugar, vinegar and red meat. Eat plenty of dark green and orange vegetables.

SUPPLEMENTS
Ginkgo Plus containing potassium ascorbate and bilberry to improve micro circulation.
GLA is an essential fatty acid which increases blood flow by reducing stickiness in red blood cells. Citrase, a supplement made from magnesium and calcium which aids circulation. BC

HINTS
Massage your feet with diluted essential oil of Black Pepper or Rosemary which will help improve circulation and increase blood supply. Regular reflexology improves circulation.
Magnet Therapy - Use Magnet Insoles known to improve circulation. For details call 01942 840188 or contact Nikken UK, Unit 7, Landmere Lane, Edwalton, Nottingham NG12 4DE. Tel: 01159 456595.
Sixtan Anti Cold Foot Balm based on alpine herbs and herbal extracts to increase circulation. Available by mail order from JICA Beauty products Ltd, 20 Island Farm Avenue, Molesey Trading Estate, West Molesey, Surrey KT8 2UZ or call 0181-979 7261.
Keep on the move and get plenty of exercise, especially in cold weather.

CHRONIC FATIGUE (see Exhaustion and ME)

CIRCULATION (see also Raynauds)

Circulation problems usually manifest themselves in the hands and feet. Bad circulation can lead to memory loss and has been associated with conditions such as senile dementia. Bad circulation is one of the commonest problems I have dealt with. Over 25% of my letters have been from people suffering with circulatory related problems. It would appear that many of us simply could do with a lot more exercise! Bad circulation has a knock on effect throughout the body's systems which can play havoc with overall health. Tingling feet, cramps, leg ulcers are all associated with bad circulation as are many skin disorders.

DIET
Good wholefood diet, low in saturated animal fats and salt. Include one tablespoon of extra virgin olive oil every day in your diet and oily fish at least twice a week. Drink at least six glasses of filtered water every day. See General Health Hints.

SUPPLEMENTS
A bioflavinoid complex containing ginkgo biloba and bilberry extract which improves micro circulation, called Ginkgo Plus. BioMagnesium taken regularly also helps circulation.
Vitamin E, 200iu daily. Vitamin C with Bioflavonoids to strengthen capillaries. BC

Foil, a concentrated fish lipid capsule which thins the blood. FSC

Garlic is very helpful for thinning the blood- take 1 tablet like Kwai daily, or include plenty of fresh garlic in your diet.

HINTS
Take a walk every day for at least thirty minutes. Any exercise that pounds the feet gently will help improve circulation, like dancing,

skipping and rebounding. Stop smoking. If you are overweight, try and lose some for your health's sake.

Reflexology is excellent for people who for health reasons cannot manage much exercise. See index for further details.

COLDS and FLU

The common cold can be caused by any one of at least 40 different viruses for which there is no definitive orthodox treatment.

DIET

Avoid all sugar, white flour and other refined carbohydrates and dairy products which are mucous forming. Eat plenty of fresh fruit and vegetables. Avoid being in stuffy, smoky rooms for too long. Get plenty of exercise and fresh air. Avoid physical contact with anyone who has a cold or flu. Wash your hands regularly. Drink plenty of filtered water to help the body eliminate the poisons more easily.

If you get a sore throat then immediately gargle with Tea Tree Oil, a natural antiseptic. Mix 3-6 drops with warm water and gargle twice daily (Do not swallow). Also, finely chop a half inch piece of fresh ginger, stand in boiling water for fifteen minutes with lemon juice and freshly chopped spring onions, strain and sip. At the onset of symptoms take one gram of vitamin C straight away and keep repeating every two hours. Stay in one temperature for at least 48 hours until symptoms subside. Rest is essential if you have a temperature.

SUPPLEMENTS

Beta Carotene to boost the immune system.

Echinacea to help drain the lymphatic system and fight viral infections. Take plenty of Vitamin C at least 2 grams a day plus a good liquid gel capsule Multi-Vitamin/Mineral and a B Complex supplement. FSC

Muccolyte 3 times daily to help clear congestion plus garlic. BC

READING
Colds and Flu by Penny Davenport. £3.99. Element Books.
Colds and Flu by Charles B Inlander and Cynthia K Moran. £3.99.
Thorsons.

COLD SORES

Cold sores are caused by the Herpes Simplex virus which lies
dormant until activated by sudden exposure to hot or cold weather,
sunlight or viral infections. Low immune systems or stress can
trigger an eruption.

DIET
Avoid nuts, chocolates and seeds for a month as they contain
arginine an amino acid which the virus thrives upon. Eat plenty of
wholegrain cereals, low fat dairy produce, fish, fruit and vegetables
which help resist infection. Some readers have found that dairy
products made from cow's milk can trigger an attack. Use soya or
rice milk instead.

SUPPLEMENTS
1,000 mg of the amino acid Lysine taken daily helps to starve the
virus.
Liquid Bio-A drops. A potent, easily absorbed form of vitamin A.
One drop daily in liquid. Histazyme. A natural anti-
viral/inflammatory supplement. One gram of Vitamin C daily .
Derma C Cream applied topically at the first sign of any sores
forming. BC

There is a coldsore topical treatment available from Britannia
Health called Vybrit. This is herbal based with anti-viral properties
available from most health shops. Their information line is 01737
773304.

HINTS
Make sure you change your toothbrush regularly as this can carry the virus. Pierce a Vitamin E capsule and apply directly to the sores.

COELIAC DISEASE
A disorder of the small bowel associated with malabsorption of food and accompanied by small intestinal lining damage and sensitivity to dietary gluten. Most patients have suffered with this condition from childhood and there is evidence that this condition is inherited. The basis of treatment is the removal of gluten from the diet.

DIET
Avoid any products containing wheat, rye, barley and oats. Cow's milk intolerance is quite common so eliminate dairy products. Try soya products instead. Avoid sugar based foods.

SUPPLEMENTS
Glutenzyme assists in the breaking down of gluten in the body. BC Green Multi helps to replace nutrients that are not being absorbed properly. Bromelain aids digestion. FSC
Cold Pressed Evening Primrose oil. 1000mg daily to calm the system. Vitamin C Complex with bioflavonoids helps reduce bowel reaction.

READING
Diets to Help Gluten and Wheat Allergy by Rita Greer. £2.99.
Thorsons.

HINTS
Trufree Foods can supply a range of suitable flours for preparing a range of foods, plus dietary advice. Further information available from 0181-874 1130.

CONSTIPATION, BLOATING AND FLATULENCE

Some of the most common causes of constipation are drug based laxatives, long term use of which make the bowel lazy, as well as long term use of antibiotics, steroids, anti-depressants and painkillers. Digestive problems, lack of exercise and a sedentary lifestyle can also induce this condition. Inadequate fluid intake often leads to dehydration, a major cause of constipation. A very common cause of bloating is overgrowth of Candida or other unhealthy organisms in the gut (see also Candida).

DIET

Avoid bread and cereals containing wheat, as wheat bran is definitely not recommended, oat bran is better. We all know that if you mix flour and water together it makes a glue like paste, and it does the same in the bowel! Melted cheese looks delicious, but once cold it bends like plastic, again this is what happens in the bowel, so eliminate full fat cheeses, especially when cooked. Avoid cow's milk products, use soya or rice milk instead. Also avoid beef and pork. If you have a juicer, try a blend of cabbage, spinach, celery and lemon juice. Avoid too much tea and coffee which dehydrate the bowel. Make sure you drink at least one litre of bottled or filtered water every day.

SUPPLEMENTS

Colon Care until normal movement is restored.
Bio-Acidophilus twice daily to replace the good bacteria in the gut.
Sea Plasma. Excellent nutrition and great de-toxifier.
200-400mg Magnesium for one month. BC

Stabilised Aloe Vera juice has been found helpful for many sufferers. For further details call the Aloe Vera Centre in London on 0181-871 5083.

Obbekjaer's Peppermint Capsules are helpful for wind and bloating. Nature's Best make a supplement Ido-Air especially to help with bloating and flatulence. Linusit Gold Linseeds, for general health and to keep the bowel moving. Start with two teaspoons daily on food, gradually increase to one tablespoon daily with plenty of water.

READING
Food Combining in 30 Days by Kathryn Marsden. £4.99. Thorsons.

HINTS
Take a brisk thirty minute walk every day or some other form of regular exercise, especially tummy exercise which helps to stimulate the bowel. When you feel the need to pass a motion, be sure not to ignore the signal, and take the time to read a magazine on the loo! It really does help. Never bear down and strain as this causes piles and increases the risk of varicose veins.

CRAMPS
A painful muscular spasm or contraction, often caused by poor blood supply to the muscles. Cramps can occasionally be due to a deficiency of salt, but this is quite rare. Do not increase salt intake unless excessive exercise and sweating are involved. Cramp is more commonly caused by a lack of magnesium or calcium as well as bad posture.

DIET
Lots of potassium from fruit, especially bananas and naturally sodium rich foods like celery and fresh vegetables. Nuts and seeds will give you much needed magnesium. Reduce coffee, tea and highly spiced foods.

SUPPLEMENTS
Ginkgo Plus, containing potassium ascorbate, ginkgo and bilberry helps the circulation. BC
Super Multi Mineral Complex, containing calcium and magnesium which usually relieve cramp, plus Vitamin E 200iu. FSC

HINTS
A regime of regular exercise is beneficial like walking, swimming or yoga. Regular massage of the feet and legs whilst raised will also help to improve circulation. See a chiropractor or try reflexology. See index for further details.

CROHN'S DISEASE

An inflammatory disease which tends to affect multiple areas of the intestine and produces a thickening of the bowel wall. Symptoms include weight loss, loss of appetite, diarrhoea, fever and malabsorption of nutrients from food. Other areas of the body can also become inflamed. Crohn's sufferers are often found to have a poor diet.

DIET

Avoid foods that cause bad reactions, the most common being dairy products made from cow's milk, wheat, oats, rye, barley, corn and any products which contain white flour and sugar. Sweeteners that contain fructose or sorbitol seem to be a problem. Consider food combining which will help take the stress off your digestive system.

SUPPLEMENTS

Gastroplex capsules with each meal have been shown to aid digestion together with Liquid Multi-Vitamins which are easily absorbed. BC

Slippery Elm is helpful, but use only the pure powder. Mix three grams of Slippery Elm with two grams of Peppermint Powder in a glass of purified water and drink fifteen minutes before meals. Take Acidophilus capsules twice daily to replace the good bacteria in the gut, along with a Magnesium Compound for cramps. B12 and Bio-Zinc 1 daily of each, together with a Calcium Compound to help absorption of nutrients from food. BLK

READING

The Complete Guide to Digestive Health by K Mayes. £4.99. Thorsons.
How to Improve Digestion and Absorption by C Scarfe. £2.50. ION Press.

HINTS

Crohn's Disease is exacerbated by stress, therefore any techniques that help to reduce stress should prove helpful such as yoga, meditation, massage or hypnotherapy. Adequate rest is essential for any Crohn's sufferer and gentle exercise is also beneficial.

For further help contact The National Association for Colitis and Crohn's Disease (NACC),98a London Road, St Albans, Hertfordshire AL1 1NX.

Crohn's in Childhood Research Association (CICRA) Parkgate House, 356 West Barnes Lane, Motspur Park, Surrey KT3 6NB.

CYSTITIS

Cystitis is a painful inflammation of the bladder. Symptoms include the urge to urinate and a burning sensation when passing water. If you have blood in your urine, you may have a kidney infection and should see your doctor.

DIET
Avoid products containing yeast and sugar like bread, cakes, biscuits and soft drinks. Also avoid vinegar, soy sauce, mushrooms and alcohol, which also contain yeast and sugar. Drink at least six glasses of water and eat a live organic low fat yoghurt every day.

SUPPLEMENTS
Bio-Flavonoids at least 2 daily during an attack.
UR228 Uritol Capsules and CP227 Cystoplex, made from cranberries which contain hippuric acid to prevent bacteria clinging to the bladder wall. Two grams of Vitamin C daily as an anti-inflammatory. Cervagyn Cream can be applied topically to ease the itching. BC

READING
Bladder Problems By Rosy Reynolds. £3-99. Thorsons.
Cystitis:Prevention & Treatment by Angela Kilmartin. £4.99. Thorsons.

Cystitis Information Sheet. Send 4 first class stamps to Green Library, 9 Rickett Street, London SW6 1RU or call 0171-385 0012.

HINTS
Sometimes caused by sexual intercourse which creates friction and forces an infection into the bladder. Try and use the loo after intercourse and drink a glass of water. Avoid perfumed soaps and vaginal deodorants. Wear cotton underwear. Avoid tight fitting jeans, especially in hot weather. Douche daily with diluted Tea Tree Oil or add a few drops to your bath. Acupuncture and homeopathy have helped many sufferers. See index for details.

DEPRESSION

Typical symptoms of depression are unhappiness, irritability, pessimism, fatigue, insomnia, headache, anxiety, loss of sex drive, fearfulness, and suicidal tendencies. It can also lead to lack of concentration and difficulty in making decisions.

DIET
Avoid all junk and sugary foods, alcohol and caffeine which can cause severe mood swings. Keep your diet as healthy as possible by eating plenty of fresh vegetables and fruit. Depression can also be caused by food allergies (see Allergies). People on extremely low fat diets who have low cholesterol levels have been found to suffer from depression. Make sure that you eat the right kind of fats like olive oil, as cholesterol plays a vital role in making hormones.

SUPPLEMENTS
Vitamin B6 50-75mg plus a B Complex to support the nervous system. Niacinamide 500mg to help keep calm. One Super Multi-vitamin plus 2 grams of vitamin C and Magnesium daily. FSC DLPA (an amino acid) has proved helpful. LGF

People with depression have reported significant improvement when taking the herb St John's Wort. In tablet form it is available from the Nutri Centre on 0171 436 5122. Also try using Essential Oil of Geranium and lavender in your bath to aid relaxation.

READING
You Can't Afford The Luxury Of A Negative Thought by Peter McWilliams & John-Roger. £8.99. Thorsons.
Overcoming Depression by Dr Caroline Shreeve. £5.99. Thorsons.
How to Stop Worrying and Start Living by Dale Carnegie. £5.99. Cedar.
Mental Illness-Not All In The Mind, a very useful booklet edited by Patrick Holford which explains how diet and lack of the correct nutrients can cause depression. £1.25. To order call the Institute for Optimum Nutrition on 0181 877 9993.
How To Heal Depression by Dr H Bloomfield £7.99 Thorsons.

HINTS
Regular exercise diverts the mind, increases blood flow to the brain, and promotes positive thinking. Learn to breath properly by practising yoga. Visualisation has been successful in relieving depression during clinical trials in America. Recent studies show that counselling and problem solving sessions proved more useful than anti-depressant drugs. (Read Volume 6 No1 and No 6 of 'What Doctors Don't Tell You'. To order telephone 0171 354 4592.
For details of a counsellor in your area contact the British Association for Counselling (BAC), 1, Regent Place, Rugby CV21 2PJ Tel 01788 578328.
Many readers have found Hypnotherapy very helpful for chronic depression. See index for further details.

DIABETES
Diabetes Mellitus, commonly known as diabetes, is caused when the body produces little or no insulin, the hormone produced by the pancreas needed to transform carbohydrates into energy. Obesity can sometimes bring on diabetes, but a large number of people actually inherit the tendency for the condition. Symptoms

include being thirsty, passing a lot of urine, tiredness and sometimes coma. There are certain conditions which cannot be legally treated by alternative practitioners, diabetes is one of them. The best course of action would be to ask your own GP to refer you to a nutritionist who is also a medical doctor who can prescribe vitamins, supplements and dietary changes to suit your needs. See index for details.

DIET
There are certain guidelines that may prove helpful with your doctor's approval. Avoid all foods and drinks containing sugar. Cut out alcohol, caffeine, chocolates, salt and saturated fats like those found in red meat. Replace full fat milk with skimmed milk products or use soya milk which is non dairy, low fat and sugar free. (Check labels carefully to make sure sugar free is mentioned). Eat plenty of wholegrain cereals like porridge, wholemeal bread, brown rice, whole wheat pasta and vegetables as lightly cooked as possible, especially root vegetables. Replace animal fats with mono unsaturated fat such as extra virgin olive oil and use Vitaquell spread on your bread. Eat several evenly spaced small meals daily to keep blood sugar levels regulated.

SUPPLEMENTS
Supplements found helpful in recent trials are niacin and biotin, which are found in B Complex vitamins. Chromium is helpful for controlling blood sugar levels, but can only be taken under medical supervision, and zinc is essential for insulin secretion. Try Cantassium's GTF Chromium and B3, and Zinc Complex. Also Vitamin C with Bioflavonoids, Vitamin E 400 iu, plus Fish Oil Capsules, Garlic and Lecithin Granules, all taken daily have proved beneficial to some sufferers. LGF

READING
Victory Over Diabetes by Philpot and Kalita. £9.99. Available from ION tel 0181 877 9993.

HINTS

Always let practitioners know you are diabetic. Regular eye checks and foot care are also recommended as both can be affected in diabetes. Reflexology has proved very helpful for circulation. See index for further details. Regular exercise is vital when treating diabetes as it can reduce the need for insulin. Try walking for at least 15 minutes, increasing to 30 minutes daily or more.

DIVERTICULITIS

An infection of little pouches of waste matter that frequently form in the colon of middle-aged and elderly people. These pouches form as a result of lack of roughage in the diet. Diverticulitis is similar to irritable bowel which causes pain, bloating, gas, painful spasms, diarrhoea, bleeding and fever. The cause is generally one of constipation, so your diet needs re-balancing.

DIET

Avoid wheat and dairy products made from cow's milk. Replace with soya milk or rice milk. Stop eating refined foods such as white bread, cakes, biscuits, take always and pre-packaged meals which are full of additives, salt and sugar. Avoid red meats and all saturated fats, use olive oil and fish oils instead. Wheat bran often irritates the colon so use oat bran and cereals instead. Eat lots of garlic which helps combat infection. Eat live yoghurt every day. Gradually increase your intake of fibre rich foods like vegetables, brown rice, millet, pulses and fruit. Drink six glasses of filtered water each day (use a filter like Kenwood Crystal Fridge Water Filter, available from all large health shops and chemists). Use extra virgin olive oil for your salad dressing. Avoid meat and all yeast based foods like Marmite, Bovril, cheese, soy sauce and mushrooms. Concentrated sweeteners that contain fructose and sorbitol may need to be eliminated as both have been found to cause a range of digestive problems in certain people. Carageenan is a milk protein stabiliser often used in ice cream that creates a problem for many sufferers.

SUPPLEMENTS

Slippery Elm soothes sensitive digestive tracts, add one teaspoon of powder to half a cup of water, simmer for 15 minutes, cool and drink.

One teaspoon of Linusit Gold linseeds on your cereal daily, increasing to one tablespoon a day.

Aloe Vera juice has curative properties and has proved helpful with many internal problems. Start by taking two tablespoons daily increasing to four tablespoons. For details call 0181-871 5083.

Liquid Gel Multi-Vitamin containing E and B vitamins which are easily absorbed plus Folic Acid 1-2mg. Vitamin A 10,000 iu daily to help healing of damage tissue until symptoms ease. Calcium and Magnesium may also be needed due to poor absorption in sufferers. Cal Mag Citrate. FSC

READING

The Irritable Bowel Diet Book by Rosemary Nicol. £5.99. Sheldon Press.

Irritable Bowel Syndrome by Nigel Howard. £3.99. Element Books.

Irritable Bowel and Diverticulosis by Shirley Trickett. £5.99. Thorsons.

Beat IBS Through Diet by Maryon Stewart & Dr Alan Stewart. £8.99. Vermilion.

DIZZY SPELLS (see also Low Blood Sugar, Low Blood Pressure and Vertigo)

EAR ACHE (see also Tinnitus and Vertigo)

Ear ache is usually due either to an infection in the canal going down to the ear drum or an infection of the middle ear. Children under the age of five are particularly prone to ear infections which can be caused by sensitivity to certain foods such as corn, peanuts, cow's milk and wheat. If you are able to identify the culprit foods, the ear problems usually clear up.

DIET
Try replacing cow's milk with goat's milk or soya products which can be found in all good health stores. Avoid refined foods, especially sugary or salty items. Eat a good balanced wholefood diet high in fresh salads, fruits and vegetables.

SUPPLEMENTS
The continuous use of antibiotics destroy not only the infection but also the good bacteria in the gut which helps digestion and supports the immune system. To replace the good bacteria, add a quarter of a teaspoon of Acidobifidus powder to food or drink daily for four weeks. From then on include a live low-fat yoghurt every day (if your child is not sensitive to dairy) or continue with the powder three times a week.
A new natural alternative to antibiotics and which does not destroy the good bacteria, is a liquid extract from grapefruit seed called Citricidal. Use two or five drops twice daily in juice to help the child through the infection and a few drops can be diluted and placed in the ear on cotton wool. HN

An excellent hypo-allergenic chewable multi-vitamin for children is Animal Fun by Natural Flow, together with zinc and evening primrose oil. LGF

HINTS
Do not let a child swim underwater if the ears are infected.
There is a new allergy test developed by an American laboratory which is 95% accurate. For a free Allergy Factsheet, call Higher Nature on 01435 882880.
See a cranial osteopath to check the alignment of the head and neck, as misalignment can cause ear ache. See index for details.

ECZEMA

Many readers have written to me about this very distressing complaint which is an inflammatory disorder of the skin. It is usually related to allergic conditions such as hayfever, urticaria and asthma. It affects babies from about four months of age and can occur at any time in childhood or adult life. The condition varies greatly from time to time and may be aggravated by heat, cold and certain foods.

DIET

Keep to a diet full of fresh salads, fruits and vegetables; organic when possible as it is necessary to avoid all food additives, colourings and refined foods generally. Most common food sensitivities are due to dairy products made from cows milk, peanuts, potatoes, eggs, red meat and some types of fish. Drink plenty of filtered water or low sodium mineral water (see Allergies).

SUPPLEMENTS

Mega GLA or Evening Primrose Oil along with Vitamin C with bio-flavonoids. which have a natural anti-inflammatory effect.
Children's B-Complex (as these are more easily absorbed).
Liquid Bio-A. One drop daily in juice to help the skin. NC

Zinc 30-60mg is essential for healing. Take daily until condition improves.
Nature's Plus Magnesium 200mg plus a good hypoallergenic multi-vitamin Cantamega 2000
Digestive enzymes with Hcl (Hydrochloric acid) may also be particularly helpful as incomplete digestion of foods can lead to allergic reactions. (Not to be taken by people who have stomach ulcers) 1-2 with main meal for an adult. Children would need professional advice. LGF

Aloe Vera taken internally and used topically has been found helpful for eczema. The Aloe Vera Centre on 0181-871 5083.
Mr Donal Walsh DHM, MSHI founded the Cherryfield Clinic in 1986. His herbal preparations which are taken internally and used externally have proved extremely successful in treating skin

conditions. For further details contact the Hale Clinic on 0171 631 0156.

READING
Superskin by Kathryn Marsden. £6.99. Thorsons.
Aloe Vera - The Natural Healer by Paul Hornsey-Pennell. £7.95.
Order from the Aloe Vera Centre on 0181-871 5083
Eczema & Psoriasis by Stephen Terrass. £4.99. Thorsons.

HINTS
If an allergy to some food is suspected, then avoid the offending food. Avoid soaps and soap powders, use soap substitutes available from chemists.

For further help contact The National Eczema Society, 4 Tavistock Place, London WC1H 9RA.
Try Angry Skin Soother which is good when the skin is unbearably itchy and sore. It is based on juniper, cedar and other herbal extracts and is very soothing. Contact The Organic Product Company, 6 Clements Road, Ilford, Essex. IGI IBA. 0181 478 1062.

Chinese herbs have proved exceptionally helpful in many cases but you need to see qualified Chinese Herbalist and may need to have liver function checked before and during treatment. See index for details.

ELECTRICAL STRESS AND POLLUTION
Sixty years ago hardly any household owned a radio, never mind a television, computer, micro wave, portable phone or electric blanket. In a very short space of time we have made a world in which we are daily being bombarded by a dangerous enemy. Electrical pollution is one of the fastest growing causes of many major diseases. It took scientists thirty years to discover that long term exposure to X-ray machines could cause cancer, and only recently have they started to realise what electricity can do to the

human body. The sun remains our most important electromagnetic energy source and over exposure is well known to cause cancer. Night and day these electromagnetic rays pass through the delicate cells of our bodies, which were not genetically made to withstand such influences. Every time you turn on a light switch, your brain's rhythms immediately change. People who live near power lines and sub stations, and whose homes are full of electrical equipment, seem to be more prone to illnesses like ME (chronic fatigue), cancers, migraines and insomnia. Research has also shown that if there is subterranean water under a home, then this can also compound the problems because water carries an electrical charge.

READING
Electro-Pollution. How to Protect Yourself Against It by Roger Coghill. £5-99. To order call 0171 436 5122. Well worth reading for anyone who wants to know more about this subject.

HINTS
The Harmony Balance Centre sell Transend Cards on which are imprinted holograms programmed to enhance the energy of the body and give some protection from electrical stress. Also they make bottles of special crystals which harmonise the environment and protect against electrical and geopathic stresses (radiation which comes up from faults underground). For further details of the cards and harmony bottles, send a large SAE to Jacqui Beacon, The Harmony Balance Centre PO Box 3912. London NW11 6AZ.

The Coghill Research Laboratories have invented a small, easy to use, instrument called The Coghill Fieldmouse (£58-75), which tells you if you are in a high electrical energy atmosphere. For details send a large SAE to Coghill Research. Lower Race, Gwent. NP4 5UF.

Have your home dowsed by an expert if you are worried about suffering from over exposure from electricity. Send an SAE to The British Society of Dowsers. Sycamore Barn, Tamley Lane, Hastingleigh, Ashford, Kent. TN25 5HW. Tel 01233 750253.

EXHAUSTION (See also ME)

When we are exhausted, it seems that there is no escape from the daily spiral of stress which makes us feel worse. In order to escape from this dilemma, it is essential to have a complete rest. One good night's sleep and a few extra vitamins are not sufficient help once the body is totally exhausted. If at all possible take a few days off and have a complete rest. Total exhaustion is cumulative and the immune system becomes less and less effective, until you get sick or stressed out and have to stop. Take at least one hour every day to call your own. Try meditating (see Meditation), or have a warm bath with a few added drops of lavender oil. Go out for a leisurely walk. If you find it hard to sleep because you are over tired, then try to set aside one morning a week when you can have a lay in to help re-charge your batteries instead of laying awake worrying about getting no sleep! (See Insomnia). Low blood sugar is a common cause of fluctuating energy levels and food cravings. (See Low Blood Sugar.)

DIET

Avoid stimulants like coffee, tea, cola, sugar and chocolate. Sugar based junk foods lower the immune system and deplete energy levels. Keep to a healthy diet which includes plenty of live food like fruit, vegetables which give you more energy. Refuse to eat late at night, especially heavy rich foods like red meat and protein which take a long time to digest. You are better off eating complex carbohydrates at night such as vegetables and whole grains as these have a more calming effect.

SUPPLEMENTS

A high quality Antioxidant Multi Vitamin Formula, plus CoQ10 to help energy levels, both by Pharma Nord. For details tel 0800 591756.
Vitamin C, 2 grams daily to help boost the immune system.
Pantothenic acid (B5) 500-100mg
Siberian Ginseng 1000mg known as an energy booster
Magnesium 200-600 mg a day (stress lowers magnesium levels).
High Potency B Complex tablets to help stress levels. FSC

READING
All Day Energy by Kathryn Marsden. £5.99. Bantam.
Energise Yourself by Vera Peiffer. £5.99. Thorsons.
Tired All The Time by Dr Alan Stewart. £7-99. Optima.

HINTS
A good quality herbal tonic like Matol which many readers have credited with raising their energy levels. For information send an SAE to: Blue Lake Health & Nutrition, Tara, Llanmaes, Llanwit Major, South Glamorgan CF6 9XR.

EYE PROBLEMS (see also Blephartis.)
The eye is less than 2% of our body weight, but uses up to 25% of the body's nutrients. Supplements necessary for healthy eyes are vitamin C, beta carotene, vitamin E, bilberry, zinc and selenium. Avoid excessive exposure to sunlight which can cause cataracts.

EYE PROBLEMS - DRY ITCHY EYES
Red itchy eyes can be due to an infection like conjunctivitis. Allergies like hayfever, or exposure to a smoky atmosphere can cause eye irritation. Dry, itchy red eyes can also be caused by extreme tiredness. Get some sleep! Anyone with difficulty focusing should have their eyes tested and eye pain or discomfort should always be referred to a doctor.

DIET
Eat plenty of green and yellow vegetables and fresh produce in your diet, especially broccoli, and carrots (organic when possible), which are rich in beta carotene to help the eyes.

SUPPLEMENTS
Dry eyes and tear ducts can sometimes be a symptom of a lack of vitamin A,C and E. Natural Flow's Super C Complex is an excellent vitamin C formula and their Mega-Multi provides a range of nutrients including vitamin A and others necessary for eye health or

go for a more specific formula such as Cantassium's Ocutrien or SePowder. LGF

Bilberry extract is an excellent herb used to treat poor vision, cataracts and support eye tissue, made by Solgar.

HINTS
Eyebright herb can be made into a tea and when cooled, used as an eye lotion. In tablet form it is available from Natural Flow as Eyebright Extra. It has anti-inflammatory, astringent and anti-catarrhal properties. The homeopathic version of Eyebright, Euphrasia, can be used for bathing the eyes and is very soothing. Use Euphrasia Mother Tincture about four times a day using a disposable eye bath. Most good health shops should be able to order this; or call 0181 874 1130. Don't use anyone else's face cloth or towel just in case the problem is catching. If your eyes are inflamed Chloride Compound is useful to reduce redness around the eyes. For details call 01753 683815. Camomile tea is very soothing and helps reduce redness. Make an infusion with the tea bags, when cooled place on the eyes for fifteen minutes.

EYE PROBLEMS - OPTIC NEURITIS
An inflammation of the optic nerve in the eye which can cause partial or complete loss of vision which comes on over a few hours or days. May be accompanied by a pain in the eye. This is often associated with MS and can be a symptom of this condition.

DIET
Try cutting out alcohol and caffeine which can interfere with blood circulation to the eye.

SUPPLEMENTS
Bioflavonoids with ginkgo biloba are known to improve the integrity of the blood capillaries and strengthen the tissues of the eyes. Liquid Vitamin A is helpful for eye problems, 1 drop daily in juice. BioGuard Forte contains beta carotene, selenium and vitamin E, 1 daily. BC

You may need large amounts of vitamin C for this condition, therefore see a nutritionist. See index for further details.

EYE PROBLEMS - PUFFY EYES

A common cause of this problem is an allergic reaction either to something you are eating regularly or to an external allergen like the house dust mite, spray perfumes, paint etc. See a kinesiologist who can determine the exact causes of the allergy which you can then avoid. It can also be a sign of poor lymph circulation or kidney weakness. (See Allergies).

DIET
Avoid tea, coffee, colas and salt as these encourage water retention, also avoid junk foods until you see the kinesiologist. Drink at least one litre of filtered water each day.

SUPPLEMENTS
Digestive Enzyme supplements with Hcl (Hydrochloric acid) may be helpful if problems are food related, but not if you have stomach ulcers. A multi-vitamin tablet like Femforte. Celery Seed Extract and Potassium Ascorbates help drainage. BC

HINTS
Manual Lymph Drainage (MLD) can also aid this condition. See index for further details. Make an infusion with camomile tea bags and when cool apply to the eyes.

EYE PROBLEMS - RED RIMMED EYES
Persistently red rimmed eyes can actually be a sign of malnutrition and lack of vitamin B. It can be a sign that your body is not absorbing all the nutrients it needs from your diet due to poor digestion. Take a vitamin B supplement daily, along with a multi-vitamin and a digestive enzyme with all main meals which will aid absorption. If your eyes are inflamed, take an anti-inflammatory mineral supplement like Chloride Compound which helps reduce

redness. For details call 01753 683815. Bathe the eyes in cooled camomile tea which is very soothing. See General Health Hints.

FATIGUE (see Exhaustion)

FIBROIDS

The growth of fibroids seems to be related to a hormone imbalance and is strongly linked to a high intake of oestrogen. If you are on the pill or HRT, both of which contain synthetic oestrogen, you may wish to discuss coming off these drugs with your GP, in order to help prevent further growth. Always consult a doctor if you have very heavy periods, painful intercourse and bladder or bowel pressure.

DIET

There are certain foods which contain compounds to help regulate oestrogen levels, the most potent being broccoli and soya products, as well as cabbage, Brussels sprouts, and cauliflower. Eat these vegetables raw to maximise their effect or make fresh vegetable juice daily and drink immediately. Regular intake of linseeds (like Linusit Gold from health Shops), contains a substance called Lignin which helps to balance hormone levels. Reduce all animal fats and increase your intake of fibre which helps to reduce the production of oestrogen.

SUPPLEMENTS.

Start taking at least one gram of Vitamin C daily along with 200iu of Vitamin E and a multi-vitamin. The herb Dong Quai is well known for its balancing effects on hormonal levels. LGF
There is also evidence to show that a regular intake of bioflavonoids and beta carotene can help this condition.

READING
Balancing Hormones Naturally by K Neil. £4.95. Available from ION.
Call 0181 877 9993.

HINTS
There is now a natural alternative to HRT made from wild yams.
This new supplement has been found useful for reducing fibroids.
For details see under menopause.

FLATULENCE (see also Constipation)
Caused by an excessive amount of gas in the stomach or in the
lower intestines. It may be due to swallowing air, fizzy drinks, and
certain foods like wheat and cow's milk which regularly cause
digestive problems. There are also several medical problems that
can bring on flatulence; partial blockage of the intestine, problems
with acid and indigestion in the stomach, gallbladder disease or
hiatus hernia. One of the most common causes of flatulence is
excessive fermentation in the gut due to over growth of yeast or
other unhealthy organisms. If the symptoms are persistent or
severe, see your doctor.

DIET
Certain foods especially pulses, beans, cabbage, Jerusalem
artichokes, onions, and garlic can cause flatulence in some people.
Chewing foods well and not hurrying meals or eating excessively at
any one meal will help. Food combining is known to help alleviate
this problem. In the case of pulses, soak them overnight and
discard the water; then boil them in fresh water along with a strip of
Kombu seaweed; this can help to reduce flatulence by breaking
down the enzymes in the beans. Include fresh ginger in your diet
which stimulates gastric juices and aids proper digestion.

SUPPLEMENTS
Phytozyme, a digestive aid with each meal. For three months take
Bio-Acidophilus twice daily to replenish good bacteria in the gut,
which aids digestion. BC

Many readers report that a product made from Slippery Elm, Meadowsweet and Liquorice called Natraleze is a natural remedy for indigestion. £4.09 for 60 tablets from chemists and health food stores.

HINTS
Chronic flatulence can also be a symptom of food intolerance, irritable bowel syndrome, candida or gut infections. If you are concerned, see a qualified nutritionist. See index for details.

FLU (see Colds)

FOOT PROBLEMS
I have received a multitude of letters on foot problems, so forgive me if they are not all included here, or this would become a book about feet!

FOOT PROBLEMS - HOT BURNING FEET
Certain drugs can cause this side effect as can poor circulation (see Circulation). People suffering from diabetes often have problems with their feet. By improving circulation this condition can be improved. Believe it or not, this can also be linked to digestive problems. An acupuncturist can free the body's energy channels for you. See index for further details.

SUPPLEMENTS
This problem can also be due to vitamin B deficiency, so take a B complex daily with your main meal. See General Health Hints.

HINTS
Try using an Energy Roller, a wooden spiked roller developed over ten years by a reflexologist. It hurts a little initially, but stimulates

pressure points. Many readers have reported increased circulation. For details send an SAE to Shakti Chakra. PO Box 3984, London, SE12 0DZ.

FOOT PROBLEMS - NUMB/TINGLING FEET
If you have numb and tingling feet take the vitamins suggested under circulation. Get plenty of exercise and try reflexology to help get your circulation moving. See index for further details.

FOOT PROBLEMS - SWOLLEN FEET AND ANKLES
A recurrent circulatory problem in middle-aged women which causes great distress (See Circulation). Can also be caused by extremes of heat and cold. This may also be a symptom of heart or kidney problems. A common cause of fluid retention is food intolerance. See allergies.

Try a Silica and Sulphur compound for three months to help improve the tone of your tissues, making them less likely to become waterlogged. Sit with your feet at hip level for 15 minutes every day moving your feet back and forth to improve circulation. On days when you are feeling particularly uncomfortable, take Herbal Fluid Balance made from dandelion leaves which are a potassium rich diuretic. For details call 01753 683815.

DIET
As a potassium-sodium imbalance can aggravate this problem, avoid all junk foods which contain a lot of salt and promote swelling. Meat is high in sodium, especially red meat, so try avoiding all meat including chicken for six weeks. Include in your diet lots of potassium rich foods, especially dark green vegetables like spinach, kale and cabbage along with lots of fresh fruit. Eliminate salt completely from your cooking and do not add it to your food. Sugar attracts water so reduce sugar based foods. Drink plenty of filtered water to help elimination and take regular exercise.

SUPPLEMENTS
Celery Seed Extract , Potassium Ascorbates, are good for drainage. Plus a good multi-vitamin. BC

HINTS
If the symptoms persist after following the advice given here for more than six weeks, ask your GP for a thorough check up.

FROZEN SHOULDER
May be caused by torn muscle fibres which lead to muscle and ligaments becoming strained. Inflammation in the shoulder joint and muscle spasms in the capsule of the joint will tend to become inflamed and irritated, not to mention extremely painful.

DIET
Avoid all acid forming foods like meat, bread, cakes, biscuits and dairy. See General Health Hints.

SUPPLEMENTS
For immediate pain relief take a natural pain killer derived from Willow Bark called Salagesic available from pharmacies and health stores.

Try a supplement called Ligazyme to aid repair of the connective tissues. At least one gram of Vitamin C daily along with Mega GLA both of which are anti-inflammatory. NC

Bromelain, Turmeric and Ginger are known as effective anti-inflammatories. For details call 01204 707420.

HINTS
Ask your doctor to refer you to a chiropractor or for physiotherapy, which in many areas is available on the National Health.
Meanwhile make an ice pack by wrapping a small bag of frozen peas in a tea towel. Apply to the painful area for five minutes

several times daily. Use your local swimming pool, as gentle movement in warm water loosens the shoulder. Acupuncture may also help alleviate some of the symptoms. See index for further details.

GALLSTONES

Gallstones usually consist of a sediment of cholesterol, bilirubin and bile salts and occur in individuals with excess cholesterol in the blood or as a result of an infection in the gallbladder. The gallbladder sits under the liver and gets rid of unwanted substances such as cholesterol and billyruben into the bile duct which in turn drains into the intestine. Symptoms include, colic, sweating, vomiting, possibly jaundice and in certain cases severe abdominal pain. Gallstones affect 10% of the population over the age of 40, and are at least twice as common in women. People who are overweight have an increased risk of gallstones. Recent research has shown that many gall bladder patients suffer food allergies and once the allergen is found then surgery is often unnecessary. See Allergies.

DIET
Reduce all saturated fat intake like red meat and dairy products made from cow's milk. Try soya or rice milk instead which is non dairy, low fat, sugar free and delicious. Avoid junk foods like hamburgers which contain too much salt and sugar, along with refined carbohydrates such as bread and cakes made with white flour. Avoid fatty, fried foods and eggs, which are known to trigger gall bladder problems. Drink at least eight glasses of filtered water daily and increase intake of extra virgin olive oil, which is thought to help dissolve the stones. Add plenty of fibre to your diet, which is found in fruits, vegetables, oat bran and wholegrain cereals like porridge.

SUPPLEMENTS

Herbs like Milk Thistle are useful for stimulating bile secretion and dissolving cholesterol. Try Natures Plus Liv R Actin Milk Thistle daily with each meal. Lecithin granules increase the solubility of cholesterol and help reduce the formation of gallstones, use one tablespoon daily on your cereal. People who suffer from gallstones tend to be deficient in Vitamin C and E, so take at least one gram of Vitamin C and 400iu of Vitamin E every day. LGF

GENERAL HEALTH HINTS

• Take regular exercise to a sensible level, but never go to extremes. You will be amazed at the difference regular exercise can make to your overall well being. If you do nothing else try and walk for thirty minutes daily.

• Try to make time for breakfast. Start your day with an oat based cereal or a sugar free muesli.

• Drink at least six glasses of filtered water daily. Try not to drink too much fluid with food because it dilutes the digestive juices and pushes food too quickly through the system, which can lead to poor absorption of nutrients.

• Cut down on tea, coffee, alcohol and fizzy sugary drinks which dehydrate the bowel, whilst the additives and sugar can cause hyperactivity and mood swings.

• Aim to eat two to three pieces of fresh fruit and three portions of vegetables or salad daily. The darker green the leaves, the more nourishment. Steam vegetables when possible as boiling destroys vitamins. Wash all fruit and vegetables in filtered water to remove any residue from chemical fertilisers. Buy organic whenever possible.

• Keep food simple - say no to rich foods with rich sauces and to fried foods.

• Avoid pre-packaged, take away, and tinned foods whenever possible as they are often full of salt, sugar and additives.

• Do not add salt to your food as it can aggravate water retention and cause blood pressure to rise.

• Do not become fanatical about fad diets. Everything in moderation and keep a balance of foods at all times for good nutrition. I love cakes but try and bake them only once a week!

• Use extra virgin olive oil in cooking and salad dressings. It has tremendous health benefits, from lowering cholesterol to aiding skin problems. I take at least one tablespoon daily.

• Sit down to eat your meals; chew your food slowly to aid digestion. Help digestion further by eating fruit between meals and not as a dessert.

• Cut down on any food containing refined sugar, which has no nutritional value whatsoever and can cause hyperactivity, mood swings and depression. Avoid artificial sweeteners. If you are desperate for sugar use organic rice syrup, honey or molasses instead, found in any good health shop.

• Cow's milk is often a problem for many people. Skimmed milk is higher in sugar and many people are lactose intolerant. Try soya milk or rice milk which are non dairy. Also use sheep's or goat's products and eat plenty of live yoghurt which is rich in calcium.

• Use butter sparingly. Although butter is better when baking cakes than margarine as it does not go rancid when cooked. Use a non-hydrogenated spread like Vitaquell or Superspread, available from good health stores and supermarkets.

• Wheat based cereals, especially wheat bran seem to cause bowel problems for many people. Use oat based cereals and bran instead. Pasta seems to be well tolerated by most people.

• Try to avoid red meat which can putrify in the gut and may contain drug and hormone residues. Instead use free range chicken or fresh fish.

• Avoid smoking and being in smoked filled rooms.

• Make time for yourself to relax. Stress related disorders when the body starts pumping adrenalin ready for the 'fight or flight' syndrome, in the end leads to us blowing a fuse. It can be a gastric fuse, leading to ulcers or a heart fuse causing heart attacks etc. The body and mind are one. If you are stressed something has got to give in the end. Vitamins and diet alone will not keep you healthy. Stress is a major factor. Remember you are special - give yourself the odd treat and make space every day in your diary for yourself.

• Get plenty of fresh air and learn to breathe deeply; this aids relaxation. Deep breathing helps to alkalise the body. Stress makes it too acid. Avoid over exposure to the sun and wear a sunscreen in summer.

GENERAL SUPPLEMENTS FOR BETTER HEALTH

Supplements that I take daily as part of my health regime and accredit for my overall well-being :

Green Barley, Chlorella, Sea Plasma or Blue Green Algae. Because most of us eat too many acid forming foods such as bread, cakes, protein etc, these super rich green foods are packed with nutrients and provide an essential alkaline forming balance as well as helping to detoxify the system. They are packed with concentrated nutrients usually found in fresh vegetables in a very digestible form. They are also a rich source of protein, iron, calcium, Vitamin C, beta carotene and fibre. I take a green supplement every day and believe that this is the food of the future. Ask for details at your health store. Eat more organic broccoli, which is packed with healthy nutrients.

Aloe Vera Stabilised Juice is rich in vitamins and amino acids. Devotees say that a daily drink of this ancient plant extract is fast becoming an absolute necessity, relieving constipation, irritable bowel and indigestion, the list is endless. I take two ounces every day in fresh vegetable juice as an energy booster.

Most important of all give yourself some worth while pollution protection and give your immune system a boost by taking one gram of Vitamin C along with a good multi-vitamin + mineral. Vitamin E 100-400 iu, 10-30mg of Beta Carotene and 100-200mcg of Selenium. These levels are not available in a normal diet and are not toxic in any way. I have done this and found it to be of great benefit.

Take one acidophilus capsule daily. This helps to replenish the good bacteria in the gut and helps prevent many problems like candida, yeast infections, constipation and an over acid system caused not only by our foods but all the chemicals we ingest from the air.

Whenever I am feeling particularly tired I take Get Up and Go every morning instead of breakfast. I mix the powder which contains seeds, fibre and at least 100% of all recommended daily vitamins and minerals, with either soya or rice milk. It is a real tonic. For details call 01435 882 880.

GLANDULAR FEVER
Glandular fever is usually caused by the Epstein Bar virus and is often mistaken for flu. Symptoms include sore throat, fever, chills, swollen glands, chronic fatigue, depression and vulnerability to other infections. It is very contagious. Sometimes patients with glandular fever also develop a mild hepatitis caused by the Epstein Bar virus. Antibiotics are of no use because it is a virus. Rest and good nutrition are vital to recovery so take things easy to prevent a relapse.

DIET
Eat plenty of fresh vegetables like carrots, cabbage, broccoli, spinach and kale which are high in beta carotene and magnesium. Incorporate an adequate intake of free range poultry, fish, whole-wheat bread, brown rice and oatmeal in your diet but avoid sugar and sweetened foods and drinks, especially if you experience bloating (which may be an overgrowth of Candida Albicans, which often occurs with this condition). Drink at least six glasses of filtered water daily, use a good water filter like a Kenwood Crystal Fridge Water Filter. Avoid alcohol and smoking.

SUPPLEMENTS
Calma is magnesium in powder form, for better absorption of nutrients when we are ill. Take daily in juice as magnesium levels are usually low when a viral infection attacks the body.
Garlic for boosting the immune system and fighting infection. Selenium, to detoxify the body and combat fatigue. A Multi-Vitamin/Mineral formula. Acidophilus to aid digestion and replace

the good bacteria in the gut. Evening Primrose Oil and plenty of Vitamin C. HN

HINTS
A gradual return to normal life is necessary because over-activity too soon can cause a relapse. Check for possible iron deficiency (see your doctor) and take iron if necessary. If after two months your energy and appetite have not returned contact a qualified nutritionist. See index for further details.

GOUT

Gout is a form of arthritis which is usually caused by high levels of serum uric acid causing crystal deposits in the joints. It is common in the big toe but can also attack the kidneys and skin. Attacks may be precipitated by eating rich food, drinking too much alcohol on a regular basis, accident or trauma.

DIET
Avoid alcohol, anchovies, fatty fish, shellfish, red meat, animal fats, cheese, coffee, tea, colas and all sugary drinks and sweets which can exacerbate this condition. Stop adding salt to your meals and avoid tinned and pre-packed foods which often have a high salt content. Cherries are helpful and when in season eat up to half a pound daily. Out of season, frozen or tinned cherries can be eaten. eat copious amounts of fresh vegetables, fruits and their fresh juices. Eating a ripe pear before each meal is an old French remedy. One reader found that when he gave up malted drinks, such as Horlicks, his gout disappeared. Drink plenty of pure water to enable your kidneys to excrete as much uric acid as possible.

SUPPLEMENTS
Celery Seed extract capsules which increase the elimination of uric acid. Vitamin C as Magnesium Ascorbates, BioMagnesium, GLA an essential fatty acid and Procydin, made from the pulp of cherries,

blueberries and blackberries, which are known to be powerful antioxidants. BC

The herb Devil's Claw helps to neutralise the poisons causing the inflammation. Take daily whilst the attack lasts. Cannot be used during pregnancy. Made by Solgar available from health stores.

READING
Curing Arthritis The Drug Free Way by Margaret Hills. £4.99. Sheldon Press.
The Natural Way with Arthritis and Rheumatism by Pat Young. £3.99. Element Books.

HINTS
Do not take aspirin if taking anti-gout drugs.

HAIR LOSS
When a person is very stressed, the scalp becomes very tight resulting in restricted circulation which leads to the hair follicle becoming undernourished and the hair falling out. Hair is composed of protein and minerals, and requires a healthy balanced diet for proper nourishment. Hair loss in men is often hereditary. However, dietary supplements and massage can help slow down hair loss. Sudden hair loss in women can follow child birth and there are a number of other conditions like menopause and protein deficiency which can thin hair or make it fall out.

DIET
Stick to a well balanced diet which includes plenty of fresh fruit, vegetables and proteins like beans and pulses. Drink plenty of water, at least six large glasses daily. Some people are unable to absorb all the nutrients from their food and need to take a digestive enzyme with their daily meal. See General Health Hints.

SUPPLEMENTS
Vitamin E 300 iu and Zinc Citrate for hair and nail growth.
CT 241, based upon natural extracts of marine food, especially for hair and nails. Biotin, Folic Acid, and Vitamin B are helpful for hair growth. Acidophilus to improve digestion and absortion of nutrients. BC

READING
Coping with Sudden Hair Loss by Elizabeth Steele. £6.99. Available from Hairline International, Lyons Court, 1668 High Street, Knowle, West Midlands B93 0LY
Natural Solutions to Hair Loss and Scalp Problems by David Satchell. £4-95. Allborough Press. To Order from Action Against Alopecia. Tel/Fax. 01323 412723.

HINTS
Take regular aerobic exercise which will stimulate your heart and circulation increasing oxygen flow, reducing stress and promoting scalp and hair health. Jojoba oil rubbed into the scalp can be very helpful for removing old layers of cells and impurities which can impede growth. Massage scalp firmly for ten minutes each day to improve circulation, this really does help.
Action Against Alopecia - membership £20 per annum PO Box 2505, 3, Upperton Road. Eastbourne. East Sussex. BN21 1AA
Tel. 01323 412723.
The Institute of Trichologists 228 Stockwell Road, London SW9 9SV. 0171-924 2195.
Natural Hair Products Ltd specialise in reversing hair loss in both men and women using a holistic approach which include supplements. For details call Mr Chris Pick who is a clinical nutritionist on 01798 343 600.

HALITOSIS (Bad Breath)
See a qualified dental hygienist every six months. Use floss and mouthwash daily. Change your toothbrush regularly and clean your

teeth at least twice daily. This problem can also stem from the digestive system. Naturopaths believe that by improving digestion and bowel function, any food rotting in the gut can be removed and with it any residual odour.

DIET
Keep your diet as clean as possible by avoiding junk and sugar based foods. Also avoid red meat, full fat milk, coffee, and alcohol for a month to see if this helps. Food combining is a healthy way to eat and helps improve digestion. Smoking causes bad breath. The spice coriander is helpful for killing the bacteria, so use plenty in your cooking. See General Health Hints.

SUPPLEMENTS
Acidophilus Bifidus capsules are essential, as is Digestive Aid, a mixture of herbs and vegetable enzymes to be taken with each meal to aid digestion and absorption of nutrients. BLK

HINTS
Use a natural antiseptic mouthwash like Tea Tree Oil. Add a few drops to warm water and use as a mouthwash, but do not swallow.
With your doctor's permission have a colonic irrigation which gently washes out the upper and lower bowel. See index for further details. A colon cleansing programme available for home use by Natural Flow. For details call 0181-874 1130.

HEALING AND HEALERS

Over the years I have heard an awful lot of people express negative opinions on this subject. Many people even accuse healers of using occult practises; to be frank this is beyond ludicrous. Energy healing is a scientifically proven fact. We all have energy fields around our bodies, most commonly known as auras. These can be photographed using Kirlian photography, which show many colours indicating the state of our internal health. If we are sick, then the aura is automatically affected. Healers aim to literally place healthy energy inside you and your aura, to re-balance your system and aid healing. As in every profession, there are average healers and there are brilliant healers. Some people are born with a natural aptitude for maths or playing the piano, and are called geniuses or prodigies. Healers like Seka Nikolic and Matthew Manning, who have both been tested by scientists to measure their energy levels, were born with this energy and have gone on to fine tune and develop their ability throughout their lives.

People like me who love to give healing, but were not born with a natural aptitude can go for lessons and learn. Anyone can learn to heal people if they have a genuine desire to help and to keep an open mind.

Spiritual Healing is given by people who believe that the source of the healing energy comes from a divine origin, and they simply become a channel for this energy. Much the same way that electrical sub stations transfer electricity from the generating source to the consumer. People seeking healing should always contact a reputable organisation such as The National Federation of Spiritual Healers who will put you in touch with an accredited registered healer who has received thorough training.

READING
Dr Dan Benor is a practising psychotherapist and healer who has published more than 150 scientific studies of healing in humans and animals. Healing Research by Dr Daniel Benor. Helix Books. Volume One is £29-60 Volume Two is £22-00. To order call 01524 68765. Highly recommended for any doctor who would like to know more about healing and healers.
The Complete Healer by David Furlong. £9.99. Piatkus Books
Light Emerging, The Journey Of Personal Healing by an ex NASSA space scientist who is now a healer, Barbara Ann Brennan. £16-99. Bantam Books. To order call 0171 436 5122. Her books on healing are well worth reading.

HINTS
For information, contact The NFSH, Old Manor Farm Studio. Church Street. Sunbury on Thames. Middlesex. TW 16 6RG. Referral line for your nearest two healers call 0891 616080. For general information call 01932 783164.

HEART PROBLEMS
(See also Angina, Circulation and High Blood Pressure)

Typical symptoms of a heart attack include a severe pressing band of pain across the chest which can spread up the neck in to the jaw, or across the shoulders and down in to the arms and hands. The pain is very often associated with sweating and feeling nauseous. Immediate medical aid should be sought.

DIET
Wholefood diet rich in vegetables, fruits, grains and fresh nuts (especially walnuts) and seeds. Avoid red meats, salt and animal fats and include oily fish at least twice a week or take fish oil supplements. Include plenty of fresh garlic in your diet as it thins the blood and aids circulation.

SUPPLEMENTS
Vitamin C and the amino acid Lysine help to reverse blockages in the arteries. Vitamin E, Magnesium, B Complex, B6, Selenium, Omega 3 fish oils and Co Enzyme Q10 are all beneficial to the heart.

CH192 is a combination of enzymes that aid circulation. BioMagnesium to help with elasticity of arteries and Linseed Oil capsules to improve blood flow. BC

READING
Beat Heart Disease Without Surgery by Jillie Collings. £6.99. Thorsons.

Heart Health For Women by Felicity Smart & Dr Diana Holdright.£6.99. Thorsons.
Super Nutrition for a Healthy Heart by Patrick Holford £2.50. To order call 0181 877 9993.

HINTS
For a healthy heart, don't become overweight and take regular exercise, which not only aids the heart, but reduces stress, a major cause of heart problems. See a doctor who is also a nutritionist. See index for further details.
Contact the British Heart Foundation, SAE to 14, Fitzhardinge Street, London W1H 4DH. Tel 0171 935 0185

HEARTBURN (see Acid Stomach and Indigestion)

HIGH BLOOD PRESSURE
A common condition which occurs with increasing frequency as you get older. There certainly seems to be an inherited tendency, as many cases of high blood pressure have no obvious cause. Some people have it as secondary symptom to kidney disease or hormonal problems. If you have high blood pressure, make sure it is checked regularly.

DIET
Researchers in the Netherlands have found that mineral salts containing magnesium and potassium can help to reduce blood pressure. A drastic reduction of salt (sodium) was also found to be beneficial. Excess sodium can cause water retention which increases blood pressure. In the West we eat far too much salt, especially in instant foods. Our typical diet contains 19,000 milligrams of sodium a day but the maximum we should ingest is 3,000 milligrams. So reduce salt and sugar intake, including artificial sweeteners. Bi-carbonate of soda is mainly sodium, like table salt (Sodium Chloride) which can cause water retention and increase

blood pressure. Your diet should be low in saturated fats like red meat and high in healthier fats like extra virgin olive oil, which is ideal in salad dressings. Eat plenty of high fibre foods, like whole grains pulses, wholemeal bread, potatoes (not fried), vegetables, fruit (which are high in potassium), and for essential oils eat oily fish like mackerel at least twice a week. Cut down on any drinks which contain caffeine and alcohol. High levels of lead in your drinking water are known to contribute to hypertension, so if you live in an area with soft water buy a good water filter like a Kenwood Crystal Fridge Water Filter.

SUPPLEMENTS
Garlic with your main meal. BioMagnesium, as low levels are often found in high blood pressure sufferers. Vitamin C daily. Vitamin E 200 iu daily to protect the heart.
CH192 contains enzymes and nutrients to strengthen the heart muscles and aid circulation. BC

READING
Recipes For High Blood Pressure by Maggie Pannell. £5.99. Thorsons.
High Blood Pressure By Dr Caroline Shreeve. £4.99. Thorsons.
Hypertension. A pamphlet published by What Doctor's Don't Tell You. £2-90. To order call 0171-354 4592.
Super Nutrition for a Healthy Heart by Patrick Holford £2.50. To order call 0181 877 9993.

HINTS
Cayenne pepper is anti-hypertensive. Use one teaspoon daily in cooking. Hot but helpful! (Do not use if you suffer from stomach ulcers). Stress and anxiety play a major role in raising blood pressure as does being over weight. Learn yoga and deep breathing which will help to lower hypertension. Try Ruthmol or Vita-Salt instead of table salt, which are potassium and not sodium based. Both are available from your health shop or Ruthmol is available by mail order from Larkhall Green Farm on 0181-874 1130. Exercise is vital in controlling high blood pressure, with your doctor's permission start walking briskly for 30 minutes daily.

HYPERACTIVITY

Children and adults who have an inability to concentrate, are unable to sit still, suffer severe mood swings and are difficult to quieten down. Sleep is a major problem for hyperactive people. Almost always caused by too much sugar, food additives, and a poor diet. Also excessive exposure to neurotoxins such as lead, along with deficiencies in nutrients such as chromium and zinc can have a dramatic effect on behavioural patterns.

DIET

Diet should be low in sugar, salt and refined foods like cakes, biscuits white bread, chocolate and cola type drinks. Concentrate more on wholefoods including organic vegetables, fruits, whole grain cereals, fish and free range chicken.

SUPPLEMENTS

Zinc and a good children's multi-vitamin which must be hypoallergenic.

READING

The Allergy Survival Guide by Jane Houtton. £10.99. To order 0171-436 5122.
How to Get A Peaceful Night's Sleep by Heather Welford. £4.99. Thorsons.
The Hyperactive Child by Belinda Barnes & Irene Colquhoun. £3.50. Hyperactive Child Cookbook by Dulcie Roberts and Janet Ash. £6.50. Both from HACSG, 71 Whyke Lane, Chichester, West Sussex.
Wholefood Books, 24 Paddington Street, London Wl, have a very good stock of books on hyperactivity, allergy and nutrition.

HINTS

For further information send an SAE to The Hyperactive Children's Support Group, 71 Whyke Lane, Chichester, West Sussex PO19 2LD. 01903 725182.

INCONTINENCE (see Bladder Problems)

Inability to hold urine in the bladder is often due to lack of control of the sphincter muscle which keeps the urine in. Often called stress incontinence, because passing water occurs whenever there is any pressure on the bladder, sometimes even when you laugh or cough. I have received hundreds of letters from embarrassed women, and I have to confess that on this one, ladies, I personally resorted to surgery. I had two weeks off work, found a good gynaecologist who specialised in this surgery and had myself stitched up. I have to say that doing the Jane Fonda aerobic workout is much easier these days!

DIET
In women the problem can be hormone related, and plants containing hormone like substances may be helpful. These include soya beans and soya products and members of the cruciferous family, ie: cabbage, broccoli, and cauliflower, which are best eaten raw.

SUPPLEMENTS
A good multi-vitamin, vitamin C and magnesium with calcium to aid muscle control.

READING
Bladder Problems by Rosy Reynold. £3.99. Thorsons.

HINTS
Try using a set of vaginal cones, containing weights to help strengthen the muscles. For information on the Aquaflex System, call 0800 614086. There is also a Helpline available on 0800 526177.

Check for bladder inflammation which can also contribute to the problem. Squeeze the sphincter muscle and hold for five seconds, twenty times daily. Eliminate the possibility of food allergens which may be irritating the urethra.

Contact the Continence Foundation, 2 Doughty Street, London WC1N 2PH. This charity provides information and advice and has a

Helpline on 0191 2130050 Monday-Friday 9am-6pm.
An osteopath will be able to ensure proper alignment of bones in the pelvic area. Acupuncture has proved helpful to some readers as has Aromatherapy. See index for further details.

INDIGESTION (see also Acid Stomach and Low Stomach Acid)
A lack of nutrients or eating heavy, rich meals can often lead to indigestion, bad absorption, and abnormal reactions which include bloating, stomach infections and poor elimination. This can disrupt every system in the body. Never eat when you are stressed as the digestive system shuts down under pressure. Eat slowly, chew food thoroughly and don't over eat. Indigestion can be caused by eating foods that are too heavy and hard on the digestion like fatty red meat. Other causes range from an excess of alcohol to heavy smoking or it can be an underlying symptom of a more serious disease of the gallbladder or the stomach, ulcers or a hiatus hernia.

DIET
Fruit passes through the stomach quite quickly, but other foods like proteins and starches, take much longer. Fruit ferments, when eaten on top of a large meal producing gas and causing indigestion. Always eat fruit in between meals. Food Combining is now recognised by many doctors as an excellent way to stop indigestion. Don't eat too much in one sitting. Eat a low fat live yoghurt once a day. Avoid drinking too much with meals as this dilutes digestive secretions.

SUPPLEMENTS
Chlorella is a supplement made from concentrated sea algae. In addition to being a good source of nutrients, it is particularly rich in plant based digestive enzymes which when taken with food can help towards proper digestion and assimilation. If flatulence is particularly troublesome, or if indigestion is recurring, then take a new enzyme aid called Phytozyme with every meal. NC

Take Acidophilus daily which helps replenish good bacteria in the gut, which in turn aids the digestive process.

Ginger capsules are very useful for indigestion, 500-1000 mg as needed.

Many readers report that a product made from Slippery Elm, Meadowsweet and Liquorice called Natraleze is a safe and natural remedy for indigestion. £4-09 for 60 tablets from chemists and health food stores.

HINTS
See a nutritionist who will help to re-balance your system. See index for further details.

INSECT BITES

Research suggests that low vitamin B levels in the blood may influence the insect's choice. Take a B Complex daily. Thiamine and zinc when excreted through the body give off an odour which repels insects; but to be effective, a dosage of 100mg of thiamine three times daily, would be necessary and at least 60mg of zinc. The herb Feverfew repels insects, take daily as necessary. Otherwise try an essential oil preparation for repelling insects. Mix ten drops of lavender oil, ten drops of orange oil, five drops of eucalyptus and five drops of citronella into a base of 50mls of apricot or almond oil and use sparingly on exposed areas of skin at night. Alternatively, place a few drops of this combination onto any light bulbs in the room, as the aroma will again act as a repellent. Avoid wearing any perfumed toiletries at night and use cotton night clothes that cover the arms and wrists. Eating fresh garlic also has a natural repellent effect.

INSOMNIA (See also Sleeping Pills)

This problem affects one in five people in the UK today. I have been a chronic insomniac for nearly twenty years and I know exactly how it feels to be wide awake at 3am, worrying about having to be up and ready for work at 8am. For myself and many others the problem has always been an inability to shut down and let go of all the thoughts that are going through our minds. The simple fact is that once you are able to let go of these thoughts, sleep comes. A good way to overcome this problem is meditation, which enables you to relax and feel more peaceful (See Meditation). Sleeping pills may work in the short term, but over extended periods they begin to lose their effectiveness and actually make sleeping more difficult.

DIET

Avoid all sugar based foods and caffeine at night along with fatty foods which are hard to digest. Don't eat late at night, as digesting takes up a lot of energy and can keep you awake. Alcohol dehydrates the body and often causes you to wake in the middle of the night. Carbohydrates like pasta and potatoes are easier to digest than protein. Drink Camomile or another herbal tea before bed. If you can't sleep, don't panic. Get up, and do something relaxing like reading a book; then go back to bed. Don't try to go to sleep, let yourself fall asleep naturally.

SUPPLEMENTS

Melatonin is secreted by the pineal gland which regulates our internal body clock. It is widely used to help people overcome jet lag and to regulate sleep patterns. I found this supplement useful when I stopped taking sleeping pills. It is now available on prescription. For years Melatonin was available at health stores in a synthesised form which has an identical molecular structure to the Melatonin that is produced in our bodies. Pharmaceutical companies are now producing a Melatonin based sleeping pill which will be chemically altered. Therefore as it is now only available on prescription make sure that you fulfill your prescription from a health store that supplies natural Melatonin. Before going to bed, place one tablet under the tongue. For further details on natural Melatonin call the Nutri Centre on 0171 436 5122.

Sleeping pills deplete the body of vitamin B therefore take a B Complex every day. Many people who cannot sleep are deficient in Magnesium, Calcium and Zinc, along with Vitamin B3. FSC

READING
Restful Sleep by Deepak Chopra. £7-99. Rider.
A Good Night's Sleep. Free. Send 2 first class stamps to Green Library, 9 Rickett Street, London SW6 1RU or call 0171-385 0012.

HINTS
Many readers have found Isocones which work on pressure points helpful in aiding natural sleep. Made by Sea Bands for details call the Nutri Centre on 0171 436 5122. Reflexology, homeopathy, acupuncture and hypnotherapy have all proved useful in restoring natural sleep patterns. See index for further details. Persistant insomnia also denotes food allergies in which case it would be wise to consult a doctor who is also a nutritionist.

INTERMITTENT CLAUDICATION (see Circulation)

IRRITABLE BOWEL SYNDROME (IBS)
(See also Diverticultis)
Also known as spastic colon, IBS is a recurrent disorder in which there are bouts of mild abdominal pain with diarrhoea and sometimes constipation in an otherwise healthy person. It often results from stress or a sensitivity to certain foods like wheat or cow's milk. Keep a food and emotional stress diary to see when the attacks are worst, then you may isolate the culprit. Many people who suffer IBS also have Candida. See a qualified nutritionist who can completely re-balance your diet.

DIET
Avoid foods high in acid like citrus fruits, plums and rhubarb; also acid forming foods like red meat, sugar and salt. Eat a good wholefood diet (See General Health Hints). Fructose and sorbitol are sweeteners which affect some sufferers quite badly, so check food labels carefully.

SUPPLEMENTS
Aloe Vera Juice has been found helpful. Four ounces daily in fresh juice or a sugar free drink.

Absorption is often a problem for IBS sufferers, therefore you may not be getting enough nutrition from the food you eat, so try taking a Liquid Multi-Vitamin Complex each day. If Candida is present then Candicidin and Bio-Acidophilus are very effective. Digest Aid with meals if there is a food intolerance. NT188 containing B vitamins and herbs like Passiflora to calm the nerves. BC

Obbekjaer's Peppermint Capsules or tables from health shops is very good for a range of digestive problems including IBS. Peppermint is an anti-spasmodic herb.

READING
Aloe Vera The Natural Healer by Paul Hornsey-Pennell. £7.95. Available from the Aloe Vera Centre on 0181-871 5083.
Irritable Bowel and Diverticulosis by Shirley Trickett. £5.99. Thorsons.
Irritable Bowel Syndrome Special Diet Cookbook by Jill Davies and Ann Page-Wood. £5-99. Thorsons.
Beat IBS Through Diet by Maryon Stewart Dr Alan Stewart. £8-99. Vermilion.

HINTS
Woman's Nutritional Advisory Service 01273 487366.
Gentle exercise like yoga, swimming or walking every day helps with IBS as exercise lowers stress levels which can exacerbate the problem. A daily banana has helped many people.

KIDNEY STONES

If you suffer from persistent lower back pain near the waist line or pass blood in urine, you may have a kidney infection. The majority of kidney stones are composed of calcium oxalate. The stones occur when this substance crystallises in the kidneys.

DIET

Avoid any foods containing oxalic acid; like beetroot, cocoa, chocolate, currants, dried figs, rhubarb, parsley, spinach, tea, blackberries, gooseberries, oranges, strawberries, raspberries, carrots, green beans, onions, cucumber and lemon peel. It is wise not to take calcium supplements. Eat less animal protein, salt and sugar, as these increase urinary calcium. Take two tablespoons of virgin olive oil daily in cooking or salad dressings. Drink at least six glasses of filtered water daily, and avoid alcohol. See General Health Hints.

SUPPLEMENTS

Magnesium helps to prevent calcium depositing in the kidneys and joints, so take a daily Synergistic Magnesium along with Vitamin B6 which helps to normalise oxalic metabolism. Q

HINTS

Inactivity tends to keep calcium in the kidneys, therefore regular exercise such as swimming, walking or cycling will aid prevention of more stones forming.

LEG ULCERS (see also Circulation)

A common problem among the over 60's caused by restricted circulation and lack of oxygen and nutrients to the skin.

DIET

Increase the amount of dark green leafy vegetables in your diet such as cabbage, kale and broccoli, which contain high levels of beta carotene and vitamin K. Eat plenty of natural live yoghurt and try to eat free range poultry instead of red meat; also add fish, whole-meal bread and oatmeal. Include plenty of fresh garlic in your diet as it is anti-bacterial and aids healing (See General Health Hints).

SUPPLEMENTS
Take ten drops of Citricidal, a natural antibiotic, in water or juice daily. A Multi-Vitamin/Mineral. Zinc Citrate promotes wound healing. Omega Flax Oil is excellent for skin, as is Vitamin C and Beta Carotene. HN

HINTS
Apply Natraderm, a potent natural skin treatment, rich in vitamins E and A to the surrounding skin and ulcer. Or try Bach Rescue Remedy Cream once the skin starts to heal, from good health stores. Bathe the leg by diluting 30-50 drops of Citricidal, a natural antibiotic, into a bath or foot bath of warm water and soak for twenty minutes. HN

Raise legs above hip level when resting and move feet backwards and forwards to increase circulation in lower legs. Try and walk for at least fifteen minutes daily. Bathing your legs in alternate hot and cold water may help as this improves circulation. Many readers have found that acupuncture and reflexology improve circulation.

Magnet therapy is known to increase circulation. For details of magnetic products send an SAE to Acar-Sud, Beaver House, York Close, Byfleet, Surrey. KT14 7HN. 01932 344447.

LICHEN PLANUS
A chronic condition of the skin and mucus membrane, such as the lining of the mouth, caused by a virus. It has features in common with other skin problems like eczema and psoriasis. The sores on the skin are often localised on the wrists or lower back, but can be widespread.

DIET
Keep to a healthy diet and avoid all dairy products and cow's milk derivatives; instead use soya products and vegetable margarines like Vitaquell or SuperSpread. Avoid stimulants such as vinegar, alcohol and hot spicy foods. Also reduce or avoid apples, cherries, pineapples, mushrooms, coffee, honey, red meat, chocolate, ice-cream, sugar and sugary foods. Eat oily fish like salmon or mackerel at least twice a week along with plenty of vegetables, raw when possible.

SUPPLEMENTS
Aloe Vera Juice, four ounces daily.

Vitamin B 12, plus BioGuard Forte which contains beta carotene, selenium and vitamin E to protect and restore skin and tissues against infection and free radicals. Mega GLA, an essential fatty acid which has anti-inflammatory properties. BC

READING
Superskin by Katherine Marsden. £6-99. Thorsons.

HINTS
A rest often helps alleviate this condition, so take regular holidays.
Use washing powders and detergents suitable for sensitive skin.
Ultra violet light often brings relief, but only do this under the supervision of a dermatologist. Moderate amounts of sunshine can help too, but try to avoid direct sunlight between 11am and 3pm.

Chickweed ointment. £4.10. For details call 0171 436 5122.

Homeopathy has helped many sufferers. See index for further details.

LOW BLOOD PRESSURE (Hypotension)

Low blood pressure may induce a sense of light headedness. I have had low blood pressure for years. Apart from not standing up too quickly when I am gardening, it causes me no problems. My doctor says that lots of athletes have low blood pressure and often live longer. It is often seen following an illness and can be a sign of other medical problems like adrenal exhaustion which will make you prone to low blood pressure, fatigue and eventually total exhaustion. Adrenal exhaustion is very common in women today. If you know that you have low blood pressure and are continually exhausted see a doctor who is also a nutritionist and he can suggest specific supplements to support adrenal function. Low blood pressure is also a sign of low blood sugar. (see Low Blood Sugar). Chronic Hypotension can also be caused by anaemia, diabetic nerve damage that disrupts blood pressure controlling reflexes, internal bleeding, malnutrition or an under-active thyroid.

DIET

Nutritional deficiencies can cause the walls of blood vessels to loose elasticity, which become flabby and expand. A high-protein diet which includes baked potatoes, leafy green vegetables, soybeans, soy flour and wheat germ, helps restore elasticity to the arteries, stimulates the adrenal glands and helps normalise blood pressure. Avoid junk foods like hamburgers and do not eat too many sugary foods. Bell peppers, cabbage, citrus fruits, cucumbers, dates, onions, peas, raisins, sweet potatoes, tomatoes and whole grains are recommended. Add a little sea salt to your diet which will help raise the blood pressure.

SUPPLEMENTS

Silica tablets to restore elasticity to the vein walls.
Vitamin E starting at 100-200iu per day for a week or two and working up gradually to 1000iu daily can help normalise blood pressure. Also take one gram of vitamin C daily.
Cactus and Hawthorn Complex is a simple herbal remedy that can help low blood pressure.
Siberian Ginseng can also help normalise blood pressure. BLK

LOW BLOOD SUGAR (Hypoglycaemia)

If you suffer from low blood sugar, also known as hypoglycaemia, the main item you need to avoid is sugar. Low blood sugar is aggravated by a diet too high in refined carbohydrates like cakes, biscuits and sweets which affects the pancreas and adrenal functions. Skipping meals, fasting, yo-yo dieting, anxiety, caffeine and other stimulants can also bring on an attack. This condition can cause a huge range of symptoms, from dizziness, fainting, sweating, extreme fatigue, insomnia and palpitations. It can also be a sign of an underlying glandular illness and if it is a recurrent problem, it should be investigated. Ask your GP for a glucose tolerance test and a thorough check-up. Ask if you can be referred to a GP who is also a nutritionist in order to balance your diet.

DIET

Eat good quality protein twice a day and fibre rich unrefined carbohydrates like brown rice and wholemeal pasta, beans and lentils. Eat several small meals a day rather than three large ones, so that you don't get hungry in between meals and let your blood sugar level drop. Avoid all junk foods and sugary snacks. Snack on fruit instead. Low blood sugar can also be associated with a food allergy (see Allergies).

SUPPLEMENTS

A Multi-Vitamin/Mineral. Chromium to help sugar cravings.
Calma, a calming calcium/magnesium drink with Omega Flax Oil which combats fatigue and cravings daily on your vegetables. **HN**

READING

Low Blood Sugar by Martin L Budd. £7.99 Thorsons.
Recipes For Health: Low Blood Sugar by Maggie Budd-Martin. £6.99. Thorsons.

HINTS

Your own GP can refer you to your nearest doctor who is also nutritionist. See index for further details.

LOW STOMACH ACID

As we age, our levels of Hydrochloric acid (HCl), the acid which digests our food, often drop, and our food is no longer digested or absorbed properly, which can lead to malnutrition and problems like osteoporosis. Undigested protein putrefies in the gut causing indigestion and wind. Ironically many people who have low stomach acid - think they have too much, and start taking antacids which prolong the problem. By supplementing our diet with HCl along with a digestive enzyme tablet the situation can often be alleviated.

DIET
Eat more dark green vegetables and fresh ginger along with alkaline forming foods like fruit and millet. See General Health Hints.

SUPPLEMENTS
Betaine Hydrochloride with pepsin, but not if you have an active stomach ulcer, along with Bromelain which aids protein digestion. Acidophilus also helps to regulate digestion. FSC

HINTS
Avoid eating too fast and cut down on alcohol consumption. Do not eat proteins with carbohydrates. Have a protein and vegetable meal or a carbohydrate and vegetable meal. Meat or fish is OK with vegetables; but when you eat potatoes, rice or bread, do not mix any of these with proteins.

ME (Myalgia Encephalomyelitis)

ME is an area of controversy, because not every doctor agrees that it exists, often putting the symptoms down to depression or even laziness which makes it very hard for genuine sufferers to receive proper attention. Each case is highly individual and sufferers who have written to me find certain things that help one person, have no effect on another. It is essential to listen to your body and rest as much as possible, exertion only exacerbates the problem. Many sufferers complain of digestive problems, which may be related to Candida Albicans in the intestinal tract. See Candida.

DIET
Avoid all caffeine and alcohol. Reduce intake of sugar based and junk foods. Eat plenty of high energy foods like fruit, vegetables, whole grain cereals and quality protein at least twice a day. Cut down on fats, except for extra virgin cold pressed olive oil which is good for the liver. Some sufferers have an intolerance to cow's milk, so cut out all dairy products made from cow's milk for a month and see if it makes any difference. Use soya or rice milk and products instead which are non dairy. Drink plenty of filtered water, even if you are not thirsty.

SUPPLEMENTS
Oxy-B15 Complex (containing vitamin B15, Co Q10 and Siberian Ginseng) to aid energy levels and Magnesium EAP which is often deficient in ME patients. BC

Evening Primrose Oil and Milk Thistle help to detoxify the liver, thereby boosting the immune system. BLK

READING
Chronic Fatigue, Complete Mind & Body Programme by Deepak Chopra. £7.99.
ME Post Viral Fatigue Syndrome and How to Live With It by Dr Ann Macintyre. £7.99. From Action for ME. Tel: 0891 122976.

HINTS
Empulse is a pulse electromagnetic treatment, the setting of which is governed by an analysis of the brain's electrical activity. It is a non-invasive, non-drug based preventative treatment. Details are available from: MLD Ltd, 17 Owen Road, Diss, Norfolk IP22 3ER or call 01379 644234.

For free dietary advice and an information pack send an A4 SAE with a 50p stamp to: Action for ME, Department 146, PO Box 1302, Wells, Somerset BA5 2WE. 24hr information line 0891 122976.

Many readers have literally been cured of ME by a specialist healer called Seka Nikolic. I know Seka personally and have interviewed many people (and their Doctors) who are now free of ME thanks to Seka. At the time of going to press Seka works from The Hale Clinic, 7, Park Crescent. London WIN 3HE. Tel 0171 631 0156.

Cranial Osteopathy or Bio Cranial Osteopathy has helped many people with ME as it releases nerve endings which releases energy in the body. See index for further details.

MEDITATION

The goal of meditation is to give the brain and therefore the entire system a few minutes of total rest each day. When we are active all day our brains are in a beta (busy) state. During the quiet contemplative state induced by meditation, our brains switch to an alpha state. Doctors have proved that people who meditate regularly are less stressful, have stronger immune systems and are generally healthier. Chronic insomniacs find meditation helpful as it assists in learning to shut off the constant 'brain chatter' which keeps them awake. Unfortunately not every health authority recognises the benefits of meditation, but in certain areas if your GP thinks it would be beneficial, then lessons are available on the NHS. Further information is available from the National Transcendental Meditation Freephone Helpline on 0800 269303. Further information is available from Transcendental Meditation. Freepost, London SWI P 4YY.

READING
Teach yourself to Meditate by Eric Harrison. £7-99. Piatkus Books.

MEMORY (see also Alzheimer's and Brain)

At 46 I often forget why I started a sentence! So to all who have written to me about this problem, don't panic, you are not alone! The brain is like any other organ, it needs nourishment to work efficiently. It is also dependent on how well you absorb what you eat. If your memory does not improve within three months of trying these suggestions, see your GP.

DIET
Diets high in refined carbohydrates like shop bought cakes and biscuits can deplete the body of B vitamins, and the majority of people with memory problems are deficient in Vitamin B12 and Folic acid. New research also shows that pollutants from household chemicals, drugs, smoke, exhaust fumes and industrial pollution all affect the delicate balance of the brain and thereby our memory. Sprinkle lecithin on your breakfast, especially the kind that is high in phosphatidyl choline which helps nerve transmission and memory.

SUPPLEMENTS
Brain Food includes lots of supplements to increase memory and concentration. Hi PC Lecithin which includes Phosphatidyl Choline is good for memory and circulation. Ginkgo Biloba is known to improve micro circulation especially to the brain. Easigest with main meals to aid digestion and absorption of nutrients from food. A multi-vitamin/mineral like the Optimum Nutrition Formula which contains all the B vitamins plus Folic Acid. For details of all the above supplements and a free leaflet 'Feeding the Brain - Can Nutrients Make us Smarter?' call 01435 882880.

READING
How to Develop A Super Power Memory by Harry Lorayne. £3.99. Thorsons.

Toxic Metal Syndrome by Dr H Richard Casdorph/ Dr M. Walken. £14.20. Explains how memory can be affected by toxins. To order call 0171 436 5122.

MENOPAUSE (see also Osteoporosis)

Menopause usually occurs somewhere between the ages of 45 to 55 which marks the end of the monthly cycle. Common symptoms include hot flushes, depression, loss of libido, palpitations and tension. I do not advocate taking orthodox Hormone Replacement Therapy (HRT), because of the increased risk of hypertension, weight gain, gall bladder and liver problems, not to mention breast and endometrial cancers. HRT slows the rate of bone density loss but only while you are taking it; whereas if you were to skip for three minutes daily it could increase bone density by up to 4% a year.

DIET

Chinese and Japanese women, do not suffer with menopausal symptoms as we do in the West. This is now thought to be because they eat plenty of soya products, fresh vegetables which contain hormone regulating nutrients called isoflavones. We, on the other hand overload our bodies with synthetic hormones and additives by eating meat and produce which has been sprayed with herbicides and pesticides. These compounds, like Lindane have an oestrogen like effect. Excess intake of oestrogen which is the main ingredient in the Pill and HRT increases the risk of breast and endometrial cancers. Eat plenty of foods that help regulate hormone levels, like sage, broccoli, cabbage, kale, cauliflower, soya products, whilst avoiding too much caffeine and red meat. Include plenty of extra virgin olive oil in the diet.

SUPPLEMENTS

Agnus Castus is a traditional European herb commonly used for menopausal symptoms which can be taken in conjunction with Dong Quai. These herbs also help with excess hair on the face and body due to the menopause. BLK

Vitamin E, 400iu helps ease flushes and irritabilty. Vitamin C as Magnesium Ascorbate, Femforte, a multi-vitamin especially for women, a Calcium, Magnesium and Zinc combination. BC

Many women have found relief from hot flushes by taking Co Enzyme Q10 and sage capsules.

Menophase is a combination of vitamins, minerals and herbs that help balance hormones and aid menopausal symptoms take three daily. HN

READING

Balancing Hormones Naturally by Kate Neil. £4-95. and Natural Progesterone by Dr John Lee £12-00. To my mind Dr Lee's work is absolutely marvelous and for any woman who wants to know more about taking natural progesterone should read the above books. Both available from ION to order tel 0181 877 9993.
Sexual Chemistry by Dr Ellen Grant. £5-99. Cedar.
Menopause Without Medicine by Linda Ojeda. £4-99. Thorsons.

HINTS

Natural progesterone has been available for over twenty years in America and is currently available over the counter at health shops in America and Ireland. In the UK natural progesterone is now available on prescription. Many top gynaecologists and doctors now prefer natural progesterone to HRT. It can be used by women who for medical reasons cannot take conventional HRT. Natural progesterone has been tested for over fifteen years, and no toxic side effects have been found. It is the only supplement which will actually increase bone density. I have been taking natural progesterone instead of HRT for three years. The benefits include increased bone density, increased libido and healthier skin.

A full information pack for GP's is available from The Society of Complementary Medicine. 31, Weymouth Street. London W1N 3FJ. Bob Jacobs, who is a Naturopath and Homeopath gives regular lectures on natural progesterone and can be contacted at the above address.

This cream must be prescribed by your own doctor. For a fact sheet to show your GP, send a large SAE clearly marked 'Yam Fact Sheet', to The Nutrition Line, Burwash Common, East Sussex TN19 7LX. Prescriptions can also be filled from this address.

Sylk, a natural lubricant made from kiwi fruit with no additives is wonderful for easing vaginal dryness. Details call 0181 874 1130.

MERCURY FILLINGS

There are millions of people who have had amalgam fillings containing mercury, myself included, but it is only a small proportion who are affected. Removal of these fillings has to be done very carefully so the patient does not swallow mercury and the mercury vapour is properly handled.

DIET
Avoid chewing gum which can increase the level of mercury in your mouth.

SUPPLEMENTS
Supplements which help to de-toxify the body of mercury are Vitamin C as Magnesium Ascorbates, Zinc Ascorbate and Aminoplex, which contains methionine, cysteine and lysine, amino acids to aid detoxification of the body. Selenium 200mcg daily. BC

READING
Dentistry Without Mercury by Sam and Michael Ziff. £3.95. Probe Inc. To Order call 0171 436 5122.

Biomed Report on Amalgam Toxicity by Dr Alan Hibberd available from BioMed Publications, 16 Court Oak Grove, Harborne, Birmingham.

HINTS
For specialist help in the removal of amalgam fillings contact Jack Levenson, a leading dentist who specialises in this field. The Brompton Dental Clinic, 221, Old Brompton Road. London, SW5. Tel 0171 370 0055. A fact sheet, Poisons in The Mouth, is available at this address.

There is also a specialist blood test which shows up metal toxicity. For further details contact The British Society for Mercury Free Dentistry. No 1, Welbeck House, 62 Welbeck Street. London W1M 7HB.

MIGRAINE

A severe recurrent headache usually associated with nausea and dread of bright lights. It may be an inherited tendency.

DIET

Certain foods are known to trigger migraine attacks; especially blue cheese, port wine, chocolate, and coffee. It would appear that nearly all migraines have an allergy as the root cause (See Allergies), with wheat being the most common allergen. As we age our stomach acid levels fall, and sufficient stomach acid is crucial to being able to absorb nutrients from our food. Another effect of low stomach acid is that larger than normal food molecules are allowed to enter the bloodstream where they are treated as enemies by our immune system which can trigger a migraine reaction. Try a digestive enzyme with each meal that contains Hcl, the acid required by the stomach to improve digestion and absorption of food (not if you have stomach ulcers). Toxaemia, especially in the bowel, can result in headaches, as certain bacteria in the colon can convert tyrosine to tyramine (It is the tyramine in cheese that is thought to affect so many sufferers).

SUPPLEMENTS

Feverfew (sold as Tanacet 125) at health shops or contact The Meadow Feverfew Company, 15 Bell Meadow Road, Hook, Hampshire. Tel: 01256 761995

Evening Primrose Oil capsules 3000mg daily. The ingredients are thought to block inflammatory compounds which are involved in causing migraines. Natural Flow's Bifidophilus between meals to keep the bowels clean. Magnesium, as a deficiency is often associated with migraine. Digestive Enzyme Complex tablets help digestion reducing likelihood of allergic reaction to undigested food particles. LGF

READING

The Natural Way With Migraine by Eileen Herzberg. £3-99. Element Books.

Migraine Revolution by Dr John Mansfield £4-99. Thorsons.
Migraine Hand Book by Jenny Lewis. £ 6-99. Vermilion Press.

HINTS
Migraine is often brought on by food allergies, so keep a food diary to see if you can identify foods that bring on an attack. If this is unsuccessful, a consultation with a qualified kinesiologist is well worth while. Regular aerobic exercise has been shown to reduce migraine attacks and yoga helps reduce stress levels. Migraines can also be a symptom of spinal and neck misalignment, a qualified cranial osteopath would be able to advise you on this point. Many people have found by wearing magnet jewellery, pain is relieved. For further details and a brochure send an SAE to Acar-Sud, Beaver House, York Close, Byfleet, Surrey KT14 7HN.

Further information can be obtained from the British Migraine Association on 01932 352468 Send a large SAE to 178a, High Road, Byfleet, West Byfleet, Surrey. KT 14 7ED.

Empulse is a pulsed electromagnetic treatment, the setting of which is governed by an analysis of the brain's electrical activity. It is a non-invasive, non-drug based treatment. Further details are available from: MLD Ltd, 17 Owen Road, Diss, Norfolk IP22 3ER or call 01379 644234.

MOUTH PROBLEMS

MOUTH PROBLEMS - MOUTH ULCERS
Recurring mouth ulcers can be linked to underlying causes and usually occur when the immune system is low or when foods are eaten to which you have an allergic reaction. Many readers have found oranges and tomatoes are a problem, whilst others found that ill fitting dentures bring on an attack.

DIET
Avoid any products containing sugar or white flour. Also avoid nuts (especially peanuts), strawberries, tomatoes, pineapple and any highly acidic fruit such as plums, rhubarb, kiwi fruit and citrus fruits.

SUPPLEMENTS
Multi Vitamin daily, Vitamin C, Zinc Ascorbate, Liquid Vitamin A (Bio A) 1 drop daily in juice until the bottle is finished. BC

HINTS
Tea Tree Oil is a natural antiseptic and makes a marvellous mouthwash when a few drops are mixed with warm water.
Some readers have found that they are allergic to the material false teeth are made from, ask your dentist to test you for an allergy - use porcelain as an alternative material as this has been found to ease the discomfort. Pierce a vitamin E capsule and apply the oil to the ulcers.

MOUTH PROBLEMS - BURNING MOUTH SYNDROME
Symptoms include tongue swelling, metallic tastes, and a burning sensation in the mouth. Nitrates and added chemicals found in drinking water can cause this syndrome so try using a nitrate removing water filter like Kenwood Crystal Fridge Water Filter, available at any large chemists or health stores. Avoid toothpaste and tooth powders which contain additives, aluminium and chemicals. Use a herbal toothpaste like Blackmores or Sarakan.

SUPPLEMENTS
A deficiency of vitamin B12 can also cause these symptoms, so take a good Multi-Vitamin daily which includes B12 as well as a Multi-Mineral supplement which contains zinc. Also take 2 Acidophilus capsules daily to re-balance your whole digestive system. BLK

HINTS
Mouth problems often reflect problems in the gut and digestive systems. See a nutritionist who can re-balance your diet and suggest supplements to boost your immune system.

MOUTH PROBLEMS - CRACKED LIPS

Lips that are cracked at the side usually denote a deficiency in vitamin B2. Dry, cracking lips usually mean that you are lacking in vitamin E and essential fatty acids found in evening primrose oil. Also include more olive oil in your every day diet.

SUPPLEMENTS

A Multi-B Complex plus Vitamin C, also 200iu of Vitamin E and 1500mg of Evening Primrose Oil daily which eases the dryness in your skin. Q

Many women are also deficient in zinc which is essential if wounds are to heal, take daily for six weeks and rub vitamin E cream on the affected area. FSC

HINTS

Use a lip balm like Lobello to help keep the lips moisturised.

MULTIPLE SCLEROSIS (MS)

A progressive disease of the nervous system. It develops over many years during which time the patient experiences attacks of weakness, visual problems or loss of sensation in certain parts of the body. Dr Patrick Kingsley, one of the UK's leading researchers into MS, states that in his opinion mercury is the underlying cause of multiple sclerosis, as he has found that many of his patients have an average seven and a half times more mercury in their spinal fluid than a healthy person should have. Dr Kingsley has found that severe candida yeast infections sometimes mimic MS symptoms and are often mistaken for MS. See Candida.

DIET

Avoid any foods high in saturated fat, red meat, cow's milk, cheese, shop-bought pastries, snacks, yeast and wheat. Replace wheat with rye breads and rice oat cakes. Increase your intake of essential fatty acids such as those found in evening primrose oil and fish oils. Eat whole grain cereals, such as brown rice, buckwheat, quinoa, organic buckwheat, quinoa, organic fruit and vegetables, especially greens and use extra virgin olive oil in dressings.

SUPPLEMENTS
Certain supplements aid elimination of mercury but according to Dr Kingsley this can take up to nine months. (See under Mercury Fillings for these supplements.) Try a regime that includes supplements known to de-toxify the body such as Liquid Selenium, at least 2 grams of Vitamin C daily, plus Zinc, Magnesium EAP, Vitamin B12, reduced Glutathione, Vitamin E, B Complex, Omega 3 fish oils, and Mega GLA, an essential fatty acid. [BC]

READING
Multiple Sclerosis by Judy Graham. £9.99. Thorsons.
Multiple Sclerosis by Jan de Vries. £4.99. Mainstream.

HINTS
People on a Vegan diet often have relief from symptoms - but the diet would need to be kept up for at least two years. This is because vegan diets are rich in essential fats needed for nerve function and low in saturated fat.

For information on candida, The Practical Guide To Candida by Jane McWhirter is available by mail order from Green Library, 9 Rickett Street, Fulham, London SW6 1RU £5.75 inc p&p. This book includes a UK directory of practitioners who treat candida naturopathically.

Help and advice on MS can be obtained from Solent Multiple Sclerosis Therapy Centres on 01705 699116. Send an SAE to 56 Hewitt Road, Portsmouth PO2 0QP.

NAIL PROBLEMS

NAIL PROBLEMS - FUNGAL INFECTIONS

This problem is more likely to occur when the immune system is low.

DIET

Avoid all junk food and any products that contain sugar or yeast for at least four weeks, as these lower the immune system and slow the healing process. Iron deficiency is a common cause of nail problems. To increase iron intake include plenty of fresh fish, poultry and green leafy vegetables in the diet. As vitamin C increases iron absorption, include plenty of fruit in the diet whilst avoiding coffee and tea with a meal as these prevent iron being absorbed. Eat plenty of raw or lightly cooked, yellow and orange vegetables. Incorporate plenty of extra virgin olive oil and live yoghurt in your diet.

SUPPLEMENTS

Dab Tea Tree Oil, which is naturally antiseptic and anti-fungal, directly onto the nails. In a recent study it was found that 92% of women in the UK are deficient in zinc which is essential for healing, take daily for six weeks. Vitamin C powder and Echinacea herbal tablets make an excellent immune system booster. FSC

NAIL PROBLEMS - SPLITTING AND WHITE SPOTS

White spots usually denote a lack of zinc, if your nails are brittle and splitting you need a Calcium Magnesium and Zinc supplement. An excellent one is made by Solgar, from good health stores. It can also be caused by poor absorption of nutrients from food. Take a digestive enzyme daily along with a strong multi-mineral like Super Multi Minerals, plus essential fatty acids like Linseed Oil. FSC

HINTS

Massage olive oil or evening primrose oil regularly into the nails and cuticles which speeds the growth of nail tissue. (See above dietary advice).

NUMB AND TINGLING SENSATIONS (fingers and toes)

I receive many letters from readers who have numb and tingling toes and fingers. This may be a sign of sluggish circulation. Extremes of cold can cause numbness and tingling, as during cold weather circulation to the skin is reduced. Any conditions which reduce the circulation to nerves in the skin will produce a similar sensation. A deficiency of essential fatty acids found in oily fish and flax oil (extracted from linseeds) can cause this problem. Also a deficiency of vitamin B12 common in older people can cause tingling. Walking half an hour each day will help to get your circulation moving.

DIET
Eat more oily fish such as mackerel, herrings and salmon, all good sources of essential fatty acids. See General Health Hints.

SUPPLEMENTS
Take three teaspoons of Omega Flax Oil on salads or vegetables and a quarter teaspoon of Sublingual Vitamin B12 under your tongue every day. The Optimum Nutrition Formula includes plenty of B vitamins to help with our nerves. Hi PC Lecithin Granules sprinkled on your breakfast will help repair nerve endings. Ultra C Plus with Bioflavonoids daily will aid circulation and repair of small capillaries. HN

If after taking these supplements for six weeks you still have numb and tingling toes, see your GP.

HINTS
You can talk to a qualified nutritionist on the Nutrition Line, 0891 615522, and have a consultation by telephone.

It is also helpful to massage your hands and feet. Obviously it is easy to manage one's own hands, however if you find it difficult to massage your feet, perhaps you could get a relative or friend to do it for you. Another alternative is to bathe the hands and feet in alternate warm and cool water a couple of times a day as this will improve the circulation. Reflexology is wonderful for this type of problem. See index for further details.

OSTEOPOROSIS (see Low Stomach Acid and Menopause)

A disorder in which the bones become thin and weak due to lack of calcium and bone fabric. It usually occurs in women over the age of fifty. Women most at risk are those who are very thin and those who smoke. Causes of osteoporosis range from lack of exercise, excess animal protein in the diet, stress, low weight, alcoholism, cola type drinks to steroid hormones. A recent study in the New England Journal of Medicine stated "Women who have taken HRT for ten years or more may have a greater bone density than those who have not taken it but lose increased density rapidly when the HRT is stopped and end up with only 3.2% higher bone density than women who took nothing, HRT can only prevent osteoporosis if it is taken for the rest of these womens lives." Natural progesterone is now available on prescription in the UK. It can increase bone density, thereby avoiding osteoporosis at any age. It can be taken instead of conventional HRT. For full details see under Menopause.

DIET

Western diets are mainly based on acid forming foods like proteins and carbohydrates which force the body to compensate by withdrawing calcium from the bones to alkalise the system. Coffee, tea, fizzy drinks and all acid forming foods leach calcium from the bones, so to maintain a balance eat plenty of fresh vegetables, fruit, broccoli, kale, nuts, seeds and sea vegetables which alkalise the body.

SUPPLEMENTS

Magnesium is vital to prevent osteoporosis so take OseoFormula, a supplement formulated by Dr Alan Gaby which contains all the supplements to support bones; calcium, magnesium, zinc, vitamin D, vitamin K, vitamin C, manganese, boron, copper, silica, and betaine. FSC
Take a daily Chlorella or Green Food Supplement to keep the body alkalised.

READING

Balancing Hormones Naturally by Kate Neil £4.95 and Natural Progesterone by Dr John Lee. £12. An absolute must for anyone

who wants to come off HRT and recover from osteoporosis. To order from ION tel 0181 877 9993.
Sexual Chemistry by Dr Ellen Grant. £5.99. Cedar Publishing.
Osteoporosis Prevention and Reversal by Dr Alan Gaby. £17.99. Prima Press.
Osteoporosis by Kathleen May. £4.99. Thorsons.

HINTS
The National Osteoporosis Society
PO Box 10, Radstock, Bath BA3 3YB Tel: 01761 471771.

All aerobic and impact exercises like skipping can increase bone density. Also weight lifting exercises help to strengthen bones. Regular exercise of any description is vital to help fight osteoporosis.

PANIC ATTACKS

In Britain an estimated ten million people suffer from panic attacks. They usually occur after major life changes such as bereavement, divorce, or postnatal depression. A traumatic shock or accident can induce lack of confidence and feelings of insecurity. There is often panic associated with having a panic attack. Low blood sugar is a major cause of unexplained feelings of panic (see Low Blood Sugar).

SUPPLEMENTS
Vitamin B Complex daily helps reduce stress. NT188 contains B vitamins and passiflora to keep you calm,plus , BioMagnesium to support nerves and extra Vitamin C. BC

READING
Panic Attacks by Christine Ingram. £5.99. Thorsons.
You Can Have What You Want. £5.99. and You're Great! £7.99. by Julia Hastings. Touchstones Publications. Both are accompanied by cassette tape.

The Power is Within You. by Louise Hay. £8-99. Eden Grove Editions.

HINTS
Avoid stimulants like caffeine, sugar and alcohol which can cause severe mood swings. See General Health Hints.
Bach Flower Remedies are helpful for panic attacks. Regular exercise reduces stress and builds confidence. A regular aromatherapy message helps you to stay calm. A warm relaxing bath and sound restful sleep help does wonders to ease stress. Learn how to control the attacks, fighting them will only make them worse. Tell yourself that this is just the body's way of getting you to take care of yourself. Speak to yourself gently, as you would to comfort a child.

The Phobic Society, 4 Cheltenham Road, Chorlton-cum-Hardy M21 9QN. Tel: 0161-881 1937 is a registered charity to help with anxiety disorders, teaching self-help rather than drug related therapies. Send a SAE for further information.

First Steps to Freedom is a self-help group. For further information call their Helpline on 01926 851608.

PHOBIAS
Many readers have written in with phobias of varying kinds. Some who have a chronic fear of spiders, others who had been afraid to leave their homes for years. Whilst many people find this type of condition hard to understand, the person with the phobia is truly living a nightmare. Counselling for the whole family is often necessary.

READING
Stress Control Through Self-Hypnosis by Dr Arthur Jackson. £7.99. Piatkus.
Self-Hypnosis by Valerie Austin. £5.99. Thorsons.

HINTS

First Steps to Freedom, a self-help group with a help line 365 days a year for people with phobias. Counselling, tapes and leaflets are available. The membership fee is £7.50 per year. For further information write to First Steps to Freedom, 22 Randall Road, Kenilworth, Warwickshire or call 01926 851608.

Hypnotherapy is an excellent way to find the root cause of your problem and learn how to let it go in order to lead a normal life. See index for further details.

THE PILL

The progesterone, or minipill, is taken on a daily basis and provides contraception by thickening the mucus in the cervix and making it impenetrable to sperm. The combined pill, which can cause blood clots especially in smokers, suppresses ovulation by preventing the eggs release every month so there is no possibility of pregnancy occurring. There are risks and side effects with any pill, which can be minimised by eating a good diet and taking the right supplements. Best of all try to use natural family planning. By knowing when you ovulate you can have sex safely for the latter part of the cycle and use barrier methods (cap or condom)for the rest of the cycle. For further details contact the Natural Family Planning Centre, Birmingham Maternity Hospital, Q. E. Medical Centre, Birmingham B15 2TG.

DIET

If you are on the pill many nutrients are depleted in the body such as zinc, iron, vitamin B, especially B6 and B12, vitamin C and magnesium. These nutrient deficiencies combined with stress and an unbalanced diet will have a noticeable long term affect on the immune system and can cause depression. See General Health Hints.

SUPPLEMENTS

A good multi-vitamin such as Natural Flow Mega Multi which contains a range of nutrients including vitamin B and C, along with Nature's Plus Zinc ideally to be taken last thing at night for maximum absorption. Cantassiums Vitamin C 500mg could be taken in the evenings. LGF

READING

Optimum Nutrition by Patrick Holford £5.95 ION Press.

HINTS

If you are on the pill you should not smoke. Make sure you get plenty of exercise.

PMT/PMS (Pre-Menstrual Tension/Pre-Menstrual Syndrome)

Usually a series of symptoms that women experience just prior to the bleeding part of their cycle. These symptoms vary from depression, anxiety, aggression, lack of concentration, breast swelling to abdominal discomfort. Low blood sugar often causes this condition (see Low Blood Sugar). A lack of progesterone and too much oestrogen can also cause PMT. See under Menopause for details of a natural progesterone supplement which usually alleviates this condition.

DIET

Medical studies have shown that a diet low in fat, sugar, salt and dairy foods made from cow's milk may reduce symptoms. Use soya milk and products which are non dairy. Excess sugar can cause anxiety, irritability and depression. Cut down on caffeine and alcohol, drink herbal teas and sugar free drinks. Eat a diet high in fibre, grains, fruit and fresh vegetables. See General Health Hints.

SUPPLEMENTS

These supplements should be taken every day, not just during your period: Femforte, a multi vitamin for women, 2 daily. Mega

GLA an essential fatty acid 2 daily. B6 at least 100-400mg. Vitamin C as Magnesium Ascorbates, 2 daily, 200iu Vitamin E plus PT208 which contains agnus castus, a herb known to help PMT and Bio Magnesium. BC

READING
The Pre-Menstrual Syndrome by Caroline Shreeve. £4.99. Thorsons. Beat PMT Through Diet by Maryon Stewart. £6.99. ION.

HINTS
If your life is stressful, it is vital to try and find some time each day to call your own, even if it is simply to soak in a warm bath for fifteen minutes. Add lavender oil to help relaxation.

PRICKLY HEAT
A rash of tiny inflamed pimples that itch, sometimes quite severely. Regular intake of vitamin C has been shown to reduce prickly heat. It is also possible that you are suffering from a food allergy which is sensitised when you go into the sun.

DIET
Try cutting out cow's milk, wheat, peanuts and coffee, although the culprits could be something quite unusual like radishes, bananas, or orange juice. Detoxify your body as much as possible by drinking lots of water and eating plenty of fresh vegetables and fruit. See General Health Hints.

SUPPLEMENTS
Ultra C Plus, which is high in bioflavonoids as well as vitamin C. Two teaspoons of Omega Flax oil on your vegetables or salad every day plus the Optimum Nutrition Formula, a balanced multi-vitamin/mineral. For details of these supplements, plus a free Allergy Fact sheet call 01435 882880.
If you are planning a vacation in the sun take 100mg of B6 regularly for 2 days before travelling.

HINTS

Many drugs cause sun sensitivity, especially strong antibiotics. Often emulsifiers and chemicals in sun screens can cause prickly heat. I use Soltan for really sensitive skins from Boots. Stay out of the mid-day sun and never allow your skin to go red. Use unperfumed bath soaps and gels when on holiday .

PROSTATE

A small gland that sits below the bladder. The prostate enlarges frequently in older men resulting in interference with the flow of urine from the bladder. Men with mild prostate symptoms often have to get up and pass urine several times at night and have difficulty starting off passing urine, or have difficulty finishing. If you feel you have a prostate problem, I cannot stress how vital it is for you to see your doctor immediately. Conditions of the prostate are now affecting more young men than ever before.

DIET

Reduce your intake of high fat dairy products, eat plenty of fresh chicken and fish. Try to eat organic foods, as new research shows a link between pesticide residues and prostate enlargement. Studies show that a zinc deficiency can be related to an enlarged prostate, so eat lots of pumpkin seeds which are rich in zinc and fatty acids. Eat plenty of fibre, oat bran, linseeds, fruit and vegetables. See General Heath Hints.

SUPPLEMENTS

Linseed Oil Capsules and Formula 600 containing zinc, saw palmetto, African Pygeum and amino acids are very helpful for prostate conditions. FSC

READING

Prostate Problems, The Complete Guide by Jeremy Hamand. £7.99. Thorsons.

The Complete Book Of Men's Health by Dr Sarah Brewer. £9-99. Thorsons.

HINTS
To help improve circulation to the area and reduce inflammation, lie on your back, bend your knees, bring the soles of the feet together and bring the feet as close to your buttocks as possible. Relax your legs, letting knees fall outwards towards the ground. Hold this position for five minutes. Only attempt this exercise if you are fit.

Bathing the area in alternate hot and cold water for thirty seconds, repeating three times every other day to stimulate circulation. See an osteopath to check that the pelvis is not misaligned.

For further help and advice send a large SAE to :
The Prostate Help Association. Langworth, Lincoln LN3 5DF.
or
Prostate Research Campaign UK. 36 The Drive, Northwood, Middlesex HA6 1HP.

PSORIASIS
A chronic skin disease which is often inherited, characterised by patches of mildly irritated red and scaling skin. The symptoms may not appear until adulthood and they can vary greatly in severity. Sometimes the rash can disappear for long periods of time. Many doctors feel that stress triggers this condition, so any relaxation exercise, like yoga or meditation may help.

DIET
Cut out all animal fats, alcohol and eat lots of oily fish like salmon, mackerel, sardines, tuna and herrings, as well as plenty of fresh fruits. A diet low in sugar and citrus fruits is advised.

SUPPLEMENTS
Liquid Bio A drops, one drop daily in juice. Linseed Oil. Vitamin C with bioflavonoids, and Vitamin E. A Multi-Vitamin plus Zinc Citrate, all of which support and aid skin healing. `BC`

Milk Thistle is marvellous for liver cleansing and clearing the skin. `BLK`

Some doctors are now treating their patients successfully with Aloe Vera Gel. For details call the Aloe Vera Centre on 0181-871 5083.

Cherryfields Clinic specialise in herbal remedies which can be taken internally and used externally. Their preparations have had excellent results. For further information contact the Hale Clinic on 0171 631 0156.

READING
Superskin by Kathryn Marsden. £5.99. Thorsons.
Beat Psoriasis by Sandra Gibbons. £7.99. Thorsons.
Aloe Vera, The Natural Healer by Paul Hornsey-Pennell. £7.95. To order call 0181 871 5083.

HINTS
Sea bathing is beneficial for psoriasis. Many sufferers find relief after bathing in Dead Sea Salt, because of its high mineral contents. Add 2lbs to your bath and soak for ten minutes. Moderate sun exposure also helps psoriasis.

RAYNAUD'S DISEASE
Raynaud's is an intermittent spasm of the small arteries in the fingers and toes, usually associated with exposure to cold. The digits tend to turn white and numb and then, as the spasm finishes and the blood rushes back in, they become red and usually painful depending on the severity of the spasm. Sometimes the skin can

actually ulcerate if it is starved of blood for too long. Vitamin B12 deficiency is known to exacerbate this problem.

DIET

Ensure an adequate intake of iron from lean red meat, poultry, fish, leafy green vegetables (especially broccoli) and complex carbohydrates, like potatoes, wholemeal bread, pasta, oat based cereals and seeds. Avoid drinking tea and coffee as this inhibits iron absorption as does smoking.

SUPPLEMENTS

Ginkgo Plus contains bilberry and potassium ascorbate to aid circulation. Mega GLA is a vital essential fatty acid known to aid this condition plus Lipoplex, Bio-Magnesium ,Vitamin E 100iu and Manganese. BC

A rapidly absorbable, sublingual (dissolved under the tongue) form of Vitamin B12 is available for those who find it difficult or impractical to have regular B12 injections. NC

HINTS

Take regular exercise, as this will aid circulation. Swimming, skipping and re-bounding on a mini trampoline are all wonderful ways to improve circulation.

Try wearing magnet insoles in your shoes which aid circulation. For further information contact Nikken UK, Unit 7, Landmere Lane, Edwalton, Nottingham NG12 4DE.

Try massaging hands and toes regularly with diluted oil of black pepper and rosemary. Reflexology and acupuncture have helped many sufferers. See index for further details.

For further information and advice contact: The Raynaud's and Scleroderma Association, 112 Crewe Road, Alsager, Cheshire ST7 2JA.

REPETITIVE STRAIN INJURY (RSI)

This is a nerve compression condition caused by the swelling of a ligament which presses on the median nerve in the carpal tunnel of the wrist. The patient may wake at night with a tingling pain in the hand which can be eased by hanging the hand out of the bed. The condition can be aggravated by excessive use of the wrist which should be avoided.

DIET
See General Health Hints

SUPPLEMENTS
Vitamin C as Magnesium Ascorbates. Ligazyme, optimum nutrition for the musculo-skeletal system. Colleginase strengthens connective tissue. B Complex including 200-400mg of B6. BC

HINTS
Magnets can help relieve localised pain. For details send an SAE to Acar-Sud Distribution, Beaver House, York Close, Byfleet, Surrey KT145 7HN.

Derma C Cream. Massage in after warm shower, cover with cloth to avoid staining clothes until absorbed. BC

If your work involves long hours at a computer screen, then the Ergo Rest will place your arm in the right position helping to help and reduce muscle fatigue and pain in the neck. For further details send a large SAE to Incoms Systems, Rowan House, 9-31 Victoria Road. Park Royal. London NW10 6DP. 0181-838 0077.

RESTLESS LEGS

Also known as Ekbom's Syndrome, symptoms include aching, tickling, burning or twitching in the muscles of the legs, which occurs particularly at night or when sitting still for long periods. It is particularly common in pregnant and middle-aged women, smokers, and those who drink lots of caffeine. Also commonly found in people who are deficient in iron.

DIET
Avoid all caffeine drinks like cola, tea and coffee and do not eat late at night. Eat a diet rich in nuts, seeds, avocado, green leafy vegetables, fish and poultry. Smoking is not advisable. See General Health Hints.

SUPPLEMENTS
Folic Acid daily which aids iron absorption from food, at least 1-5 mg daily. Vitamin E at least 200iu daily, Bio-Magnesium plus Mega GLA, an essential fatty acid which helps circulation and is anti imflamatory. Multi-vitamin-mineral, plus a B Complex, along with Ginkgo plus which improves circulation. BC

HINTS
Get plenty of exercise. Massage your legs using downward kneading movements from the knee to the ankle. The legs can be bathed in alternate hot and cold water to improve circulation. Try reflexology, acupuncture or regular massage to pep up the circulation. Take all the suggested supplements for at least three months.

ROSACEA

A chronic flushing condition of the skin usually found in middle-aged people. The tendency to flush can be inherited or related to emotional stress, tension, menopause, climatic conditions such as bright sunshine or certain foods and drink, especially alcohol and spicy foods. It has also been linked to the digestive system not working properly.

DIET
Avoid junk and sugar based foods as well as dairy products made from cow's milk and cheese. Use goat's, sheep's or soya milk, yoghurt and cheese instead. Eat plenty of fresh fruit and vegetables. Drink at least six glasses of filtered water every day. Avoid coffee, tea, colas, alcohol, very hot drinks and spicy foods

that often cause flushing. A combination of papaya, pineapple and orange juice or tomato, cucumber and radish juice helps to balance the skin lubricating sebum. Drink all fresh fruit and vegetable juices, immediately upon juicing whilst all the enzymes are 'live' and vitamins are at their highest concentration. New research indicates the tremendous benefits of eating raw vegetables regularly particularly cabbage, broccoli, cauliflower and spinach. These contain chemicals which help modulate hormone levels and improve the liver's detoxification function.

SUPPLEMENTS
Take one gram of vitamin C with bioflavonoids, which strengthen the tiny blood vessels. B Supreme daily, as sufferers are often low in B vitamins plus Betaine Hydrochloride (stomach acid). Ninety percent of Rosacea sufferers have low stomach acid which may be the basis of the problem. Note: Caution for those who suffer from ulcers, Hcl supplements could aggravate the condition. Acidophilus daily on an empty stomach to replenish good flora in the gut plus a Liquid Gel Multi Vitamin capsule which is easily absorbed. FSC

READING
Superskin by Kathryn Marsden £5.99. Thorsons.

SCIATICA
Sciatica is usually a symptom of a structural problem in the lower back, where the nerve is pinched as it emerges from the spinal column and runs down the back of the leg. The pain is sometimes accompanied by numbness or tingling.

DIET
Avoid coffee which inhibits the body's ability to cope with pain. See General Health Hints.

SUPPLEMENTS
NT188 contains vitamin B and passiflora to calm the nerves, plus Magnesium Malate to relax nerve endings. BC
DLPA is an amino acid which helps the body deal with pain.
Vitamin C at least two grams daily which has an anti-inflammatory effect as does Mega GLA, an essential fatty acid. NC

HINTS
When sleeping or resting, lie on your side with a pillow between your knees to minimise pelvic strain.

To reduce pain and discomfort, prepare an icepack and a hot water bottle wrapped in a towel. Place each alternatively on the site of the pain for 10 minutes and repeat, this should be done twice daily.

Try osteopathy, a chiropractor or acupuncture for further relief.

SHINGLES
A recurrence of the chicken pox virus that most of us had when we were young. The virus lives on in the spinal nerves and simply reactivates. It typically affects the trunk of the body or the face and only ever occurs on one side of the body. The pain is variable, but can be intense. The nervous system needs help when shingles takes a hold.

DIET
Increase daily intake of Vitamin C found in fresh fruit, vegetables, kiwi fruit and strawberries. Avoid chocolate, carob and nuts which worsen the condition. Eat more meat, which contains lysine known to starve the virus. Avoid all refined carbohydrates like white bread, shop bought cakes, biscuits and soft drinks which are often high in sugar.

SUPPLEMENTS
Liquid Vitamin A one drop daily in juice plus GLA an essential fatty

acid. A Multi-Vitamin/Mineral, Vitamin E, and Ginkgo Biloba. `BC` The amino acid Lysine starves the virus, take at least two grams daily, plus two grams of vitamin C daily whilst the attack lasts.

The herb Hypericum, commonly known as St John's Wort, has proved helpful for the itching associated with shingles, as it is anti-viral and helps soothe nerve endings which are often irritated. `BLK`

READING
Superskin by Kathryn Marsden. £6-99. Thorsons.

HINTS
Vitamin E oil capsules pierced and applied the sores may give some relief. Vitamin B12 injections on a regular basis have helped many people.

SINUS PROBLEMS
(see Allergic Rhinitis, Allergies and Catarrh.)

SLEEPING PILLS (Addiction - see also Insomnia)
Taking drugs over a long time period not only causes addiction but can make the insomnia worse as the delicate chemical balance of the brain becomes dependant on the drugs to carry on functioning normally. To avoid withdrawal symptoms see your GP who can prescribe a gradual lessening of your drugs on a weekly basis. Take a natural herbal remedy like Formula Z which is derived from valerian and wild lettuce, herbs proved to aid restful sleep and relaxation. (For details call 01204 707420.) Natural remedies may not work for the first two weeks due to the toxic residue in your liver left over from the drugs. Remember it takes at least one month to kick a habit or addiction, therefore be patient with yourself.

SUPPLEMENTS

Take a detoxifying agent like Milk Thistle capsules twice daily with food, or Dandelion Tea with plenty of water to help cleanse the liver for at least six weeks.

Also drink plenty of fresh vegetable juices especially beetroot which is very cleansing. Recent research in America has found that Niacinamide (Vitamin B3) helps to ease anxiety and in some cases relieves insomnia. Because the benzodiazepine family of sleeping pills replicate the action of niacinamide (a naturally occurring nutrient in the brain), this substance helps induce sleep. Try taking 500mg- 1000mg 45 minutes before retiring. Take a supplement of Calcium, Magnesium and Zinc which is often deficient in people who wake during the night. **FSC** Positive Nutrition is an amino acid formula which helps you to get over addiction to sleeping pills. For details call 01435 882880.

READING

They Said I Was Dead by Anne McManus. A personal story of how to cope and come through addiction. Available from Scarlet Press, 5 Montague Road, London E8 2HN. £8.99.

Escape From Tranquillisers and Sleeping Pills by Larry Neild £4.99 Escape From Valium and Escape From Sleeping Pills, two leaflets also by Larry Neild £1 each. Available from Escape From Tranquillisers, PO Box 20, Liverpool L17 6DS.

SMOKING

It is imperative you make a firm resolution that you actually want to stop smoking. Telephone Helplines for smokers who need support: England 0171-487 3000. Scotland 0800 848484. Wales 0345 697500. Northern Ireland 01232 663281. If all else fails, try dipping the end of your cigarette into Tobacco Pass Powder. Researched and developed in Japan, this powder helps convert 80% of the nicotine into nicotinic acid (Vitamin B3 complex) and filters out much of the tar. For details call Human Nature on 0171-328 5452. Smoking deprives the skin of oxygen, and various chemicals can dehydrate and damage cells which leads to early ageing. Studies have shown that the skin of a 40 year old who smokes is comparable with a 65 year old non-smoker, so to help yourself stay young, give up!

DIET
Eat lots of green vegetables especially broccoli, see General Health Hints.

SUPPLEMENTS
For smokers and passive smokers it is vital to ensure a regular intake of the antioxidant nutrients, beta carotene, C, E, zinc and selenium. Vitamin B is also essential for the nervous system which can be damaged by smoke inhalation. Try Natural Flow's Mega Multi daily which includes all these vitamins. Also take zinc for six weeks plus vitamin E to aid the immune system and protect cells from more damage. LGF

READING
Stop Smoking for Good by Robert Brynin. £4-99 Hodder and Stoughton.

HINTS
Traditional Herbals make a Smokers Tea to help people through a nicotine craving. Made from crushed Lobelia leaves which Mexican Indians used to chew as a tobacco substitute, the tea is available from health stores, or by mail order from Wild Oats in London on 0171-229 1063, or try nicotine patches from all good pharmacies.

The medical herbalist Andrew Chevalier suggests this remedy: Mix one heaped teaspoon of Coltsfoot and half a teaspoon of thyme into a teapot of boiling water, cool and sip. Coltsfoot strengthens the lungs and thyme is antiseptic and healing. For details call Neal's Yard Remedies on 01865 245436.

SORE THROATS (see also Colds and Flu)

Most upper respiratory infections are viral, but some throat infections like tonsillitis are bacterial and are treated by antibiotics. These bacterial throat infections very often occur without the symptoms of a cold or respiratory infection. Repeated antibiotics will eventually lower the entire immune system which is obviously depleted or the problem would not continue to reoccur. It is essential that you take acidophilus capsules after each course of antibiotics as they replace the good bacteria in the body. Sometimes when tonsils are removed the lymph nodes in the throat, which drain toxins from the body, can be put under extra strain.

DIET

Reduce dairy and all meat. Eat lots of fresh vegetables, especially carrots and other yellow vegetables, which are high in the antioxidant beta carotene. Soup made from fresh garlic, onion and fresh ginger in a miso stock base should help relieve a sore throat when sipped throughout the day.

SUPPLEMENTS

A Chloride Compound may be useful as it helps to clear lymphatic congestion and can relieve sore throats. A duo formula containing the herb echinacea and vitamin C called Echinacea Ace should boost the immune system, as both supplements are anti-inflammatory. You will also need to repopulate your digestive system with friendly bacteria that will have been killed off by the antibiotics, so take Acidophilus Bifidus capsules. BLK

Take a good multi-mineral vitamin supplement and suck Zinc Gluconate lozenges, to relieve the sore throat.

HINTS

Tea Tree Oil is a natural antiseptic, use diluted as a gargle but do not swallow.

STITCH

The pain from a stitch is almost certainly caused by an intestinal spasm and usually stops as soon as you cease exercising. You can keep excercising through stitch, but it's rather painful! A sedentary lifestyle, eating too few green vegetables and including too much sugar, caffeine and animal protein in the diet causes a reduction of calcium and magnesium in the body, leading to a build up of lactic acid resulting in regular attacks of muscle cramps or stitch. Take regular exercise to avoid the acids accumulating in the body. A maladjustment of the spine can also cause this problem as can your appendix, so have a thorough check-up with your doctor.

DIET
Include plenty of broccoli and dark green cabbage, spinach and kale in your diet. Make sure you drink at least six glasses of water daily.

SUPPLEMENTS
Try a good calcium-magnesium supplement like FSC Super Cal-mag to alleviate the muscle cramps. FSC

STOMACH ULCERS

If you suffer pain after taking alcohol, aspirin, coffee or fatty meals, you may have an ulcer and should consult your GP. In the last few years it has been discovered that a high percentage of people are infected with a bacteria called Helicobacter Pylori which can cause stomach and duodenal ulcers. Many people have few or no symptoms other than they suffer discomfort when under stress.

DIET
Avoid alcohol, coffee, saturated fats and aspirin, as well as dairy products made from cow's milk. Use soya products instead which are low in fat and sugar. Also avoid all foods that contain sugar - this

includes sugar based drinks. Ideally, try drinking a litre of cabbage juice every day, rich in L Glutamine which has been shown to heal peptic ulcers. Plantain bananas cooked are known to give relief. Regular intake of Manuka Honey from Tea Tree Blossom is anti-bacterial and aids ulcers. One tablespoon daily on an empty stomach before breakfast and dinner. For details call 0181 961 4410.

SUPPLEMENTS
Tinica Tonic, made from Horsetail, soothes the stomach lining and stops the bacterial growth. One dessertspoon, three times daily.
Citricidal, extracted from grapefruit seeds, also helps to kill the bacteria and acts as a natural antibiotic. Up to ten drops in juice daily, tastes rather bitter, but is effective.
Boost your immune system with Vitamin A, B, C, Zinc, Omega Flax Oil and Acidophilus. For details of all the above call 01435 882880.

Many people have found relief by taking four ounces of stabilised, organic aloe vera juice every day, available from good health stores.

SWOLLEN FEET/ANKLES
(see also Foot Problems and Water Retention)

TACHYCARDIA (Rapid Heart Beat)

Tachycardia, a sudden increase in the heart rate, is often accompanied by breathlessness, nausea, sweating and dizziness. This condition should always be checked by a doctor. To combat worrying, which only exacerbates the condition, learn how to breathe properly by taking yoga lessons. Also try meditation which teaches you how to stay calm when stressed. If you feel an attack beginning, splash your face with cold water, then lie down, close your eyes, breath deeply and slowly for a few minutes until the attack passes.

DIET

Avoid stimulants like tea, coffee, chocolate, colas, alcohol and tobacco which can bring on an attack of palpitations in people who are sensitive. Low blood sugar can trigger an attack, so resist all junk foods that contain sugar. Eat small regular meals which include pasta, potatoes, brown rice, wholemeal bread, vegetables, and fruit.

SUPPLEMENTS

Magnesium and Vitamin B have a vital role in keeping the heartbeat regular and nourishing the nervous system. Take a B Complex along with Magnesium daily. Co-enzyme Q 10 has a beneficial effect on the heart.

READING

Teach Yourself to Meditate by Eric Harrison. £7.99. Piatkus Books.
Heart Disease by Richard Thomas. £3.99. Element Books.

HINTS

Essential oil of lavender has a calming effect, so try a few drops in your bath. Try aromatherpy massage regularly which is very calming. Go for leisurely walks, breathing deeply. The digestive system shuts down when the body is under stress, so avoid eating if you are upset.

TASTE AND SMELL

Loss of taste and smell can occur frequently during upper respiratory infections or nasal congestion associated with the common cold (See Catarrh). This condition can also be caused by a lack of minerals in the body, especially zinc. Certain heart drugs cause loss of taste and smell as a side effect, so if you are taking heart medication, check with your GP to see if your medication can be changed.

SUPPLEMENTS

Histazyme which includes vitamin C and zinc, a lack of which often causes this problem. Also reduces inflammatory response to allergens and protects against infection. Selenium a vital mineral 100mcg daily. BC

HINTS

A water filter like the Kenwood Crystal Fridge Water Filter will help to eliminate metal toxins in water. See a qualified nutritionist who will help to re- balance and de-toxify your system. Homeopathy is also very useful for this condition. See index for further details.

THRUSH (see Cystitis and Candida)

THYROID

The thyroid gland produces a hormone called thyroxine which controls the rate of metabolism in the body. Too much thyroxine can cause an overactive thyroid (Hyperthyroidism). Symptoms include palpitations, sweating, loss of weight, bulging eyes, sometimes diarrhoea, dry flushing skin and menstrual disorders. A lack of thyroxine causes an underactive thyroid (hypothyroid).The entire body slows down causing tiredness, mental sluggishness, weight gain, exhaustion, headaches, muscle spasms and shortness of breath, constipation, hair loss and coarsening of the skin. One in ten women suffer thyroid problems. Medical attention must be sought for thyroid problems.

DIET
Poor digestion and absorption, a bad diet, toxins from ingested chemicals like paint, pesticides and food additives play a major part in lowering the immune system which causes thyroid problems. So keep to a really healthy diet, including plenty of organic fruit and vegetables like carrots, lettuce, alfalfa sprouts, and beetroot. See General Heath Hints.

SUPPLEMENTS
TH 207 is a nutritional supplement for the thyroid. A good Multi-vitamin/ mineral. BC

A vital nutrient for an underactive thyroid is Iodine. Kombu seaweed found in major health stores is rich in Iodine, or take a daily Kelp supplement. Other supplements known to help an underactive thyroid are zinc sulphate, selenium and the amino acid L-Tyrosine.

READING
Thyroid Problems by Patsy Westcott. £5.99. Thorsons.

HINTS
Many readers have found that taking stabilised Aloe Vera Juice has helped their overall health when suffering thyroid problems. If you have thyroid problems it would be wise to consult a doctor who is also a qualified nutritionist. Other readers have found that their thyroid function normalised after treament from a homeopath. Others who are taking the natural progesterone supplement instead of HRT have also seen improvements (see Menopause for details of natural progesterone).

TINNITUS

A constant noise, or ringing sound, in the ears. This is a common condition and causes range from exposure to loud noise, compacted wax, spinal misalignment, blocked sinuses due to infection or bad teeth. Beta Blockers and aspirin are known to lead to tinnitus as a long term side effect.

DIET
If it is a sinus problem, avoiding cow's milk, yeast, sugar and saturated fats may help. See Allergies and Catarrh.

SUPPLEMENTS
Muccolyte to clear sinuses. GLA an essential fatty acid, plus Zinc Citrate. (Tinnitus is often associated with as deficiency in zinc). Garlic with main meals and Ginkgo Biloba known to improve micro circulation. NC

READING
Self-Help For Tinnitus by Arthur White. £2.99. Thorsons.

HINTS
Have your teeth and gums checked as impacted wisdom teeth and tooth decay can cause this problem.
Cranial Osteopathy can release built-up tensions in the head and neck which often cause Tinnitus. Acupuncture has proved very beneficial to some sufferers. See index for further details.
Tinnitus Helpline for up to date research on 0345 090210 10am - 3pm Monday to Friday.

TONGUE PROBLEMS

A healthy tongue is generally moist with only a minimal white fur coating. Dryness of the tongue is usually an indication of de-hydration. The tongue is usually coated in people with poor oral hygiene or those who smoke excessively. A coating on the tongue can indicate an infection but if your doctor has ruled this out then the problem is almost certainly linked to poor digestion. It can also suggest a sluggish liver which again is related to the digestive system. A common cause of a coated tongue is Candida (see Candida).

DIET
Avoid sugar based and any junk foods. Eat plenty of fresh green vegetables that have been lightly steamed to retain their vitamin content. Avoid red meat which can putrify in the gut. Drink at least four glasses of filtered water daily.

SUPPLEMENTS
Take a course of Bio-Acidophilus which helps to replace the good bacteria in the intestinal tract and aids digestion Also take a broad spectrum digestive enzyme like Spectrumzyme with every meal which helps to break down the food and facilitates proper absorbtion of nutrients. NC
The herb Milk Thistle is an excellent liver cleanser. Take daily for six weeks. BLK
If you follow this regime, your digestive and elimination systems the problem often clears completely. See also General Health Hints.

READING
Food Combining in 30 Days by Kathryn Marsden. £4.99 Thorsons.

TONGUE PROBLEMS - GEOGRAPHICAL TONGUE
This condition is so called because the tongue often resembles a map of the world. The cause may be due to a change in hormones or a deficiency of B vitamins. Usually it disappears of its own accord, but sensitivity to certain foods can exacerbate the condition. See a kinesiologist who can determine if you have a specific allergy which could aggravate the tongue.

DIET
Avoid all spicy foods, vinegar and alcohol as they irritate the membranes of the mouth. Eat plenty of silica rich foods such as fresh vegetables and fruit.

SUPPLEMENTS
Silica Compound is the specific mineral needed for this condition.
Tea Tree Oil, a natural antiseptic, can be used as a mouthwash.
Acidophilus daily replaces the good bacteria in the gut.
A good multi-vitamin/mineral every day as well as B vitamins.
Some sufferers report an improvement after taking a garlic capsule
before breakfast every day.

TRAVEL SICKNESS

Stress, anxiety, lack of oxygen or too much food prior to travel can
often make symptoms worse. If you are travelling by car or coach do
not read while the vehicle is moving, and look towards the horizon
which helps to stabilise the balancing mechanisms in the inner ear.

DIET
Eat light meals before travel and avoid oily or fatty foods which are
hard to digest. Eat small amounts of fruit, or rice cakes.

SUPPLEMENTS
Ginger is very effective for preventing nausea and travel sickness,
so take ginger capsules two hours before travelling and again half
an hour before you leave. If you are on a long trip, take a ginger
capsule every hour on the road. The stress created by
apprehension about travel sickness can compound the symptoms.
To help prevent this, at the onset of symptoms take Magnesium
Compound every half hour before travelling. BLK

HINTS
Acupressure can help to control motion sickness, see a reflexologist
who will show you which points to treat. Or wear Sea Bands, which
work on a similar principle. Available from most chemists.

TREMORS
This condition can be genetic, in which case it is quite hard to treat. But certain supplements can help to reduce the degree of tremors. Anxiety, alcoholism or an overactive thyroid gland can increase the tremors.

DIET
Avoid any strong stimulants like alcohol, spicy foods, cola type drinks, strong tea, coffee and chocolate.

SUPPLEMENTS
GLA, an essential fatty acid taken twice daily, helps repair nerve endings. Magnesium and Calcium work together in the body to stabilise the nervous system. NC

B Vitamins are also vital for the nervous system, along with herbs like Valerian Root and Passion Flower which help to stabilise the nervous system. BLK

HINTS
Some readers have found relief by plunging the affected limb into cold water for a few minutes each day.

VARICOSE VEINS
Distorted and dilated veins usually found in the legs. Anything which slows the return of blood from the leg to the heart will aggravate this condition. Development of varicose veins is closely linked with constipation, so avoid straining which causes blood to flow into the lower half of the body. If you are overweight it will aggravate the problem. Veins are often worse after pregnancy. If anyone has varicose veins in the family, early prevention is better than trying to treat them later.

DIET
Include plenty of fruit and vegetables in your diet, especially

apricots, blackberries, cherries, rosehips and buckwheat, all of which contain rutin, a natural remedy for improving elasticity of veins. Avoid all junk foods that contain sugar and salt, as well as strong tea and coffee. Avoid all foods that take a long time to pass through the bowel like red meat and refined foods such as cakes, biscuits, and white bread.

SUPPLEMENTS
Silica is an excellent mineral for toughening up veins, try Blackmores Silica Compound daily for at least three months. Ginkgo Biloba is well known for improving circulation but make sure it is a full strength capsule like Ginkgo Forte 2000. Take plenty of Vitamin C with Bioflavoinoids, along with 500iu of Vitamin E daily, to help strengthen veins. BLK

The herb Butcher's Broom has proved very successful in helping varicose veins and haemorrhoids. By taking 500-1,000 mg per day you should see an improvement in the circulation in the lower limbs. This herb can also have a laxative effect. Made by Solgar vitamins.

Aloe Vera Juice 4 ounces daily in fresh vegetable or fruit juice.

Linseeds are excellent for bowel cleansing. Initially take a dessertspoon daily, gradually increase to one tablespoon. Drink at least six glasses of water every day.

HINTS
Get plenty of fresh air and walk for at least thirty minutes every day. If you are fit enough take plenty of aerobic exercise, skipping, dancing, swimming or rebounding.
Apply a little Vitamin E cream mixed with two drops of juniper oil topically where the skin is sore. For details call 01753 683815.
Use cold compresses to reduce swelling. Many readers have found relief through acupuncture, wearing support tights and putting their feet and legs up against a wall for at least ten minutes daily to give the legs a total rest.

VERTIGO

A sensation of dizziness and loss of balance, sometimes accompanied by nausea. It can be caused by impacted earwax, blockage of the eustation tube, or by viral infections of the balancing mechanism in the inner ear. Vertigo can also be caused by high blood pressure or too much catarrh (See Catarrh). Dizziness can also be a sign of iron deficiency or low blood sugar (see Low Blood Sugar), or low blood pressure (see also Low Blood Pressure).

DIET

Cut out cow's milk and cheese from your diet for one month. Replace them with soya products which are non-dairy. A food combining diet can be helpful. See General Health Hints.

SUPPLEMENTS

Garlic is very cleansing. One tablet daily. Ginger capsules to aid the feeling of nausea and dizziness. Ginkgo Biloba to improve circulation in the head. Vitamin C plus a Multi Vitamin/mineral. FSC

If you are anaemic take Quest Synergistic Iron, which also contains Vitamin C and B, daily. Q

HINTS

See a chiropractor or cranial osteopath to make sure your neck and spine are not misaligned as this can cause problems in the ear.
Hypnotherapy and Acupuncture has helped in some cases.
High blood pressure and Beta Blockers have been known to cause vertigo in some people and therefore you should check this with your GP if taking any drugs.

WATER RETENTION (OEDEMA)

Oedema is a very common condition which can be caused by hormone problems, HRT, high blood pressure, poor lymph drainage and certain heart conditions. It is sometimes associated with a sodium/potassium imbalance or food allergies (see Allergies). Have a check-up with your GP to rule out heart weakness or kidney disease. Many people suffer temporary water retention in extreme heat and after long haul flights.

DIET
Avoid all junk, pre-packaged and sugar based foods, especially those that contain sodium (salt). Cut down on tea, coffee, colas and salty foods like crisps. Eat a healthy diet of fresh vegetables, fruits and whole grains. Drink at least one litre of filtered or bottled water every day.

SUPPLEMENTS
Celery Seed Extract and Potassium Ascorbate aid drainage. Plus Femforte a good multi-vitamin for women. B6 daily is a good diuretic. NC

HINTS
Dandelion tea is a natural diuretic and a good source of potassium. Regular exercise like walking or swimming helps.

WEIGHT PROBLEMS

If you are suffering from weight problems, this can be caused by an under-active thyroid or by yo-yo dieting which never helps. Generally the diet needs to be changed to a more sensible one on a long term basis. A sensible way to eat is food combining. Depression often causes over eating as do other eating disorders like bulimia. If this is the case you should seek specialist help.

DIET

Eat slow releasing carbohydrates like oatmeal, darker breads and whole grains, plus lots of fresh vegetables and fruit. Avoid junk foods, especially the high salted or very fatty ones, and keep off coffee. Drink at least six glasses of water daily. See General Health Hints.

SUPPLEMENTS

Optimum Nutrition Formula for all the vitamins and minerals involved in energy production. HN

There is a supplement extracted from an Asian fruit called Garcinia Cambogia which contains hydroxycitric acid (HCA). In many tests it has shown an ability to curb appetite, reduce food intake by 10% and regulate production of fats and cholesterol. One of the most potent brands is CitriMax Forte, which also includes Manganese Ascorbate and Chromium to assist blood sugar levels which helps prevent sugar cravings. It should be taken 30 minutes before each meal as part of a healthy diet. It may take a few weeks to see results, but this is a safer way to lose weight. (Not to be taken if pregnant or anorexic). For further details call either 0171-436 5122 or 0121-433 3727.

Dandelion tea or pure root dandelion coffee are great for the liver and in studies have shown to substantially help weight loss.

READING

Weight Control by Stephen Terras. £4.99. Thorsons.
The Fats You Need to Eat by Jeannette Haase Ewin. £6.99. Thorsons.
The Bottom Line by Diana Moran. £4.99. Sidgwick & Jackson.
The Fatburner Diet by Patrick Holford. £5.95. ION. Tel 0181 877 9993.

HINTS

Often women on a low calorie intake, tend to become malnourished and when encouraged to eat healthy food more frequently, they actually lose weight. Eat as much healthy food as you like, which tends to stimulate the metabolism, thereby improving overall health and weight loss. Regular exercise is vital not only for losing weight but for overall health. Try and exercise for at least thirty minutes every day.

Oestrogen can cause weight gain and water retention if your body is low in progesterone. If you are suffering food allergies then you will not lose weight. If you think you have a hormone imbalance, call 01435 882964 and ask for a free Progesterone and Food Allergy Factsheet.

If you suffer from eating disorders and need help, send a large SAE to Anorexia and Bulimia Care. 15, Fenhurst Gate, Aughton. Lancs. L39 5ED.

Index - Useful Information and Addresses

The Alternative Health Information Bureau will send you a report on all known alternatives to help your condition. £25 For further details write to the AHIB, 12 Upper Station Road, Radlett, Hertfordshire WD7 8BX or call 01923 469495.

ACUPUNCTURE
Practitioners use fine, sterile needles inserted into specific points to regulate energy flow and restore health.

To find your nearest practitioner, send an SAE to: Council for Acupuncture. 179 Gloucester Place, London NW1 6DX.

AROMATHERAPY
The use of essential oils to improve health and wellbeing, by massage, inhalation, compresses and baths. Excellent for reducing stress and anxiety.

For a register of practitioners, send an SAE with a cheque/postal order for £2 to: International Federation of Aromatherapists. Stamford House, 2-4 Chiswick High Road, London W4 1TH. Tel: 0181-742 2605.

The International Society of Professional Aromatherapists, 82 Ashby Road, Hinckley, Leicester LE10 1SN

The Register for Qualified Aromatherapists. PO Box 6941, London N8 9HF.

ALEXANDER TECHNIQUE
Teaches you how to use your body more efficiently, have balance and poise with minimum tension in order to avoid pain, strain and injury.

To find your nearest practitioner, send an SAE to : The Society of

Teachers of Alexander Technique. 20 London House, 266 Fulham Road, London SW10 9EL. Tel: 0171 351 0828.

ALOE VERA CENTRE

If you have any problems finding good quality aloe vera juice or would like further information on the healing properties of aloe vera, send a large SAE to :The Aloe Vera Centre. Gardiner House, 3/9 Broomhill Road, London SW18 4JQ. Tel: 0181 871 5083/5084/5205.

BACH FLOWER THERAPY

A complete healing system used to treat emotional problems such as fear and hopelessness. The remedies are made from the flowers of wild plants, bushes and trees.

To find your nearest practitioner, send an SAE to: The Bach Centre Mount Vernon Ltd. Bakers Lane, Sotwell, Wallingford, Oxfordshire OX10 0PX. Tel: 01491 834678.

BIO-CRANIAL OSTEOPATHY

A gentle method of osteopathy concentrating on nerves in the head, neck and shoulders. Many readers have reported success with ME (Chronic Fatigue Syndrome) and arthritis from this therapy.

To find your nearest practitioner, send an SAE to: The International Bio-Cranial Academy. PO Box 44, Bangor, County Down BT20 3SY. Tel: 01247 270626.

CHINESE MEDICINE

The concept of restoring an uninterrupted flow of chi, the vital energy of the body.

For a register of practitioners send a large SAE and cheque/postal order for £2.50 to: Register of Traditional Chinese Medicine. 19, Trinity Road, London N2 8JJ. Tel: 0181 883 8431.

CHIROPRACTIC

Gentle manipulation to treat disorders of the joints and muscles and their effect on the nervous system.

For a register of practitioners, send a large SAE and a cheque/postal order for £2 to: The British Chiropractic Association. Equity House, 29 Whitley Street, Reading, Berkshire RG2 0EG. Tel: 01734 757557 or Freephone 0800 212618.

or send an SAE to: British Association for Applied Chiropractic. The Old Post Office, Stratton, Audley, Nr Bicester, Oxfordshire OX6 9BA. Tel: 01869 277111.

COLONIC HYDROTHERAPY
Method of cleansing the colon to gently flush away toxic waste, gas, accumulated faeces and mucus deposits. Check with your GP before undertaking this therapy.

To find your nearest practitioner, send an SAE to: Colonic International Association. 31 Eton Hall, Eton College Road, London NW3 2DE. Tel: 0171-483 1595.

or send an SAE to: The Colonic International Association. 50a Moorish Road. London SW2 4EG.

I personally take colonics twice a year from Margie Finchell in George Street, London W1. She can be contacted on 0171-935 5401.

COLOUR THERAPY
There is plenty of evidence to show that colour does affect our mood and behaviour, as different colours emit an aura of their own which our bodies absorb.

To find your nearest practitioner, send an SAE to: Hygeia College of Colour Therapy. Brook House, Avening, Tetbury, Gloucestershire GL8 8NS. Tel: 01453 832150.

One of the best colour therapists I have ever come across is Lilian Verner Bonds. Lilian, who is also a psychic, gives readings based upon colours of your choice and I have found her amazingly accurate. She can be contacted on 0181-349 3299. Lilian's book

Discover the Magic of Colour. £6.99. is published by Random House.

COUNSELLING

If you, or a member of your family, is in need of professional counselling, send an SAE to: British Association for Counselling (BAC). 1 Regent Place, Rugby CV21 2PJ. Tel 01788 578328.

CRANIAL OSTEOPATHY

Therapists use hands to release resistance in tissues, bones and fluids, often resulting in revitalisation of the system.

To find your nearest practitioner, send an SAE to: Cranial Osteopathic Association. 478 Baker Street, Enfield, Middlesex EN1 3QS. Tel: 0181 367 5561.

I personally see Kenneth Underhill who practises at the Hale Clinic in London tel 0171 631 0156.

CRYSTAL THERAPY

Crystals can both receive and transmit signals or energy. A good healer generates healing energy into a crystal which is then transferred to the patient. The crystal can then be used for healing purposes without the need for the healer to be present.

To find your nearest practitioner, send an SAE to: Affiliation of Crystal Healing Organisations. 46 Lower Green Road, Esher, Surrey KT10 8HD. Tel: 0181 398 7252.

If you would like to know more about crystal therapy, the Nutri Centre Library have many books on crystal healing. Tel: 0171 436 5122.

During my research I came across Francis Xavier, who is an expert in crystal healing. Francis is also a marvellous counsellor and spiritual healer who gives fascinating one day workshops. For further details send a large SAE to:The Celtic School of Natural Therapies, Ty

Gwella, 9, Blenhein Gardens, Magor, Gwent, Wales. NP6 3NA.

GENERAL ORGANISATIONS

If you want to know more about specific alternative therapies, the following organisations will be happy to give you advice and put you in touch with the practitioners and societies that now meet with their high standards of practice and therapy.

British Complementary Medicine Association.

39 Prestbury Road, Cheltenham, Gloucestershire GL25 2PT Tel 01242 226770.

Council for Complementary and Alternative Medicine.

179 Gloucester Place, London NW1 6DX. Tel: 0181 968 3862.

Institute of Complementary Medicine

PO Box 194, London SE16 1QZ. Tel: 0171 237 5165.

HALE CLINIC

This clinic is the largest alternative treatment centre in Europe with over 100 practitioners, many of whom are also qualified medical doctors. The Hale Clinic, 7 Park Crescent, London W1N 3HE. Tel: 0171 631 0156.

HEALING

The healer is a channel for the transfer of healing energy to the patient.

To find your nearest practitioner, send an SAE to: National Federation of Spiritual Healers. Old Manor Farm Studio, Church Street, Sunbury on Thames, Middlesex TW16 6RG. Tel: 0891 616080 (Mon to Fri 9am - 5pm).

I know there are hundreds of very able healers in the UK, but I would like to mention three whom I have personally benefitted from. Denis Sinclair specialises in bone problems, he can be contacted on 0181-450 9088. David Cunningham, who works all over the UK, can be contacted on 01932 231455. Seka Nikolic has extraordinary healing powers and specialises in helping people with ME (chronic fatigue syndrome). She works at the Hale Clinic in London. Tel: 0171-631 0156.

HERBALISM

The practice of using plants to treat disease. Treatment may be given in the form of fluid extracts, tinctures, tablets and teas.

For a register of practitioners, send a large SAE with two first class stamps to: National Institute of Medical Herbalists. 56 Longbrook Street, Exeter, Devon EX4 6AH. Tel: 01392 426022.

HOMEOPATHY

A highly effective form of alternative medicine. Practitioners prescribe remedies in the form of tablets, granules, powders or liquids.

To find your nearest practitioner, send an SAE to: Society of Homeopaths. 2 Artizan Road, Northampton NN1 4HU. Tel: 01604 21400.

or send a SAE to: The UK Homeopathic Medical Association. 6 Livingstone Road, Gravesend, Kent DA12 5DZ. Tel: 01474 560336.

To find a doctor who is also a homeopath, send an SAE to: Homeopathic Trust. 2 Powis Place, Great Ormond Street, London WC1N 3HT.

HYPNOTHERAPY

By allowing external distractions to fade, the therapy allows subjects to focus on the problem in hand and to change inappropriate behaviour, thought and feeling.

To find your nearest practitioner, send an SAE to: Central Register of Advanced Hypnotherapists. 28 Finsbury Park Road, London N4 2JX. Tel: 0171 359 6991.
or send a SAE to: The British Hypnotherapy Association. 1 Wythburn Place, London W1H 5Wl. Tel: 0171 723 4443.

or send a SAE to: The National Register of Hypnotherapists & Psychotherapists. 12 Cross Street, Nelson, Lancashire BB9 7EN. Tel: 01282 699378.

I personally see Leila Hart who uses Cell Command Therapy and Hypnotherapy to help patients. Leila treats most problems and disorders and you can contact her in central London on 0171-402 4311.

INSTITUTE FOR OPTIMUM NUTRITION
The Institute for Optimum Nutrition print a quarterly magazine which costs £1.95 a quarter, plus p&p. This booklet is packed with up to date health news and the latest research in alternative medicine. The institute also holds seminars on health and have in-house nutritionists. For details contact the Institute for Optimum Nutrition, Blades Court, Deodar Road, London SW15 2NU Tel: 0181-877 9993. Open Monday to Friday, 10am - 5pm.

IRIDOLOGY
A method of analysis rather than treatment, based on the theory that the whole body is reflected in the eyes. Using a magnifier, the practitioner examines the visible parts of the eyes to pinpoint physical weaknesses or potential areas of trouble.

To find your nearest practitioner, send an SAE to: International Association of Clinical Iridologists 853 Finchley Road, London NW1 8LX.

KINESIOLOGY
Science of testing muscle response to discover areas of impaired energy and function in the body. Kinesiology is especially useful if you think you have an allergic reaction either to a food or an external allergen.

To find your nearest practitioner, send an SAE to: The Association for Systematic Kinesiology. 39 Browns Road, Surbiton, Surrey KT5 8ST. Tel: 0181 399 3215.

MAGNOTHERAPY

Regular doses of magnetism can help boost energy levels, improve circulation and accelerate healing. Many people have also found relief from wearing magnetised jewellery and using magnetised products for pain relief.

Magnet Therapy Centres:

The Hale Clinic
7 Park Crescent, London WIN 3HE. Tel: 0171 631 0156.

The Bharti Vyas Holistic Therapy and Beauty Centre
24 Chiltern Street, London WIM IPF. Tel: 0171 486 7910.

Magnotherapy products are available from:

Nikken UK
Unit 7, Landmere Lane, Edwalton, Nottingham NG12 4DE. Tel: 0115 945 6595.

Acar Sud
Westfield House, Hampton Court Road, East Molesey, Surrey KT8 9BX. Tel: 0181 977 1699.

MANUAL LYMPHATIC DRAINAGE

A very gentle pulsing massage which helps to drain the lymph nodes thereby reducing swelling and pain that is related to the lymph tissues.

To find your nearest practitioner, send an SAE to:MLD UK. 8 Wittenham Lane, Dorchester on Thames, Oxfordshire OX10 7JW.

I found this very useful after a particularly painful dental operation. It helped reduce the bruising and swelling.

NATUROPATHY

Practitioner uses diet, osteopathy, and hydrotherapy to treat illness and help the body regain its natural balance and boost the immune system.

For a register of practitioners send a large SAE and cheque or postal order for £2.50 to: General Council and Register of Naturopaths. Frazer House, 6 Netherall Gardens, London NW3 5RR. Tel: 0171 435 8728.

I personally see a wonderful naturopath and homeopath, Bob Jacobs. If you have multiple symptoms and have run out of ideas Bob is the person to see. Telephone the Society for Complementary Medicine on 0171 436 0821.

NUTRITIONAL THERAPY

Healthcare system using individual diet and supplement programmes to enhance food assimilation, correct nutritional deficiencies, combat allergies and reduce toxic overload.

Send a large SAE plus £1 for information and a list of practitioners to: Society for the Promotion of Nutritional Therapy. PO Box 47, Heathfield, East Sussex TN21 8ZX. Tel: 01435 867007.

or send a SAE plus £2 to: CNEAT, 34 Wadham Road, London SW15 2LR.

NUTRITIONIST WHO IS ALSO A DOCTOR

You will need to be referred by your own GP who will be able to find the address of your nearest practitioner by contacting:

The British Society for Allergy & Environmental Medicine
P O Box 28, Totton, Southampton SO40 2LA.

I personally consult Dr John Briffa who is a wonderful nutritional physician. For details tel 0171 283 0105.

OSTEOPATHY

A system of healing that works on the physical structure of the body. Practitioners use manipulation massage and stretching techniques.

To find your nearest practitioner, send an SAE to: Osteopathic Information Service. P O Box 2074, Reading, Berkshire RG1 4YR. Tel: 01734 512051.

POLARITY THERAPY

A therapist will use bodywork, awareness skills, diet and polarity stretching exercises to help the body and mind heal itself naturally. A very relaxing re-balancing therapy useful for extreme stress and fatigue.

To find your nearest practitioner, send an SAE to: British Polarity Council. Monomark House, 27 Old Gloucester Street, London WC1N 3XX. Tel: 01524 67009.

REFLEXOLOGY

Works on the principle that reflex points on the hands and feet correspond to every part of the body. By working with pressure on these points, blockages in the energy pathways are released and encouraged to heal. An ideal way to boost circulation.

To find your nearest practitioner, send an SAE to: The Association of Reflexologists. 27 Old Gloucester Street, London WC1N 3XX. Tel: 01892 512612.
or send an SAE to: International Federation of Reflexologists. 78 Edridge Road, Croydon, Surrey CR0 1EF. Tel: 0181 667 9458.

READING

If you have difficulty in finding any of the recommended books, the Nutri Centre have an extensive library of self-help books and would be happy to order for you, or give assistance on specific subjects. Nutri Centre, 7 Park Crescent, London W1N 3HE. Tel: 0171-436 5122.

Here is a list of the numbers of all major publishers used in this book if you would prefer to order by mail-order:

Bantam Books. Tel: 01624 675 137.
Cedar Publishing. Tel: 01933 410511.
Element Books. Tel: 01747 851339.
Green Library. Tel: 0171 385 0012.
ION Tel: 0181 877 9993.
Optima. Tel: 01621 819600.
Thorsons. Tel: 0141 772 2281.
Touchstone Publications Ltd 01428 751007.
Waterstones. Tel: 01225 448595.

USEFUL READING
Eat Yourself Fit by Martin Felt. Headline Press. £7.99. Available from Waterstones Mail Order. Tel: 01225 448595. To my mind this is an extremely useful book for any one who has a variety of symptoms which seem to have no firm cause. Starting on page 53, Martin has formulated a questionnaire at the end of which you should begin to understand your symptoms.

Encyclopaedia of Natural Medicine by Michael Murray ND and Joseph Pizzorno ND Optima Press £15.99 Available to order from the Nutri Centre, this huge book is a must for anyone who wants comprehensive, alternative health information.

Food Combining in 30 Days by Kathryn Marsden £4.99 Thorsons. Kathryn is a brilliant nutritionist who saved her husband's life when he was given three months to live when suffering from cancer. That was ten years ago but thanks to Kathryn's wealth of knowledge thousands of people who follow food combining are now also well. Food combining is marvellous for anyone suffering digestive problems, irritable bowel, hiatus hernia or people who simply want to stay fit or lose weight.

Gentle Medicine by Angela Smyth. £10.99. Thorsons.
I have found Gentle Medicine to be an absolutely invaluable

source for alternative ideas and treatments. No family should be without this informative alternative encyclopaedia.

Here's Health Magazine £1.95
Highly alternative and informative monthly magazine about up to date findings in the alternative field. Available to order from any newsagent.

Homeopathy. A Practical Guide To Everyday Health Care by Robin Hayfield. Virgin Publishing £9.99. To order Tel: 0181 968 7554. I found this an extremely informative, easy to read book for anyone would like to know more about homeopathy.

Optimum Nutrition by Patrick Holford £5.95 ION Press. Packed with up to date ideas on nutrition and supplements. Written by one of the UK's leading nutritionists.

The New Super Nutrition by Dr Richard Passwater £5.99 to order from the Nutri Centre tel 0171 436 5122. Once I started this book I could not put it down. Brilliantly researched and highly informative with specific vitamin supplement information.

Testimony of Light by Helen Graves. £5.95. The C W Daniel Company Ltd. Available to order from Watkins Books Tel: 0171 836 2182. A magical story written by a nun about life after death. Whether you believe in life after death or not, this book makes compulsive reading.

WHAT DOCTORS DON'T TELL YOU
What Doctors Don't Tell You is a monthly newsletter packed with alternative health information; but more importantly, endless advice on the side effects of drugs. Anyone who has to take large amounts of medication should subscribe to this newsletter. £24.95 for a one year subscription, back issues are £2.90 each. For details write to What Doctors Don't Tell You, 4 Wallace Road, London N1 2PG. Tel: 0171-354 4592.

Further copies of this book are available in your local bookshop.
In case of difficulty copies can be ordered from Hazel Courteney,
Infinity Press, PO Box 4629, Edgbaston, Birmingham B15 3TW
enclosing a cheque or postal order for £6.95,
payable to Infinity Press.